THE COMPLETE GUIDE TO

# EXERCISE THERAPY

# THE COMPLETE GUIDE TO

# EXERCISE THERAPY

**Christopher M. Norris**

BLOOMSBURY

LONDON · NEW DELHI · NEW YORK · SYDNEY

**Note**
While every effort has been made to ensure that the content of this book is as technically accurate and as sound as possible, neither the author nor the publishers can accept responsibility for any injury or loss sustained as a result of the use of this material.

Published by Bloomsbury Publishing Plc
50 Bedford Square
London WC1B 3DP
www.bloomsbury.com

First edition 2013

ISBN: 978-1-4081-8226-0 (pb)
ISBN: 978-1-4081-9379-2 (epdf)
ISBN: 978-1-4081-9378-5 (epub)

A CIP catalogue record for this book is available from the British Library.

Acknowledgements
Cover photograph © Shutterstock
Inside photographs © Laura Scott-Burns with the exception of: Exercises 7.10 and 8.14 and Figures 8.3, 8.4, 12.6 and 12.7 © Grant Pritchard; and Exercises 8.8, 8.15, 10.12 and 11.7 and Figure 12.4 © Christopher M. Norris
Illustrations © David Gardner with the exception of: Figures 2.1, 3.4, 3.5, 3.6, 3.9, 3.11, 4.3, 4.9, 5.5, 12.1, 12.2, 12.3 and 12.5 © Jeff Edwards; and Figures 2.5, 3.2 and 4.2 © Jean Ashley
Commissioned by Charlotte Croft

This book is produced using paper that is made from wood grown in managed, sustainable forests. It is natural, renewable and recyclable. The logging and manufacturing processes conform to the environmental regulations of the country of origin.

Typeset in 10.75 on 14pt Adobe Caslon by Susan McIntyre

Printed and bound in China by C&C Offset Printing

10 9 8 7 6 5 4 3 2 1

# CONTENTS

# INTRODUCTION

Exercise is an essential part of treatment for most musculoskeletal conditions and/or injuries, and the use of exercise as therapy is vital during recovery – in the famous words of John Dryden, 'The wise for cure on exercise depend' (*Epistle to John Driden of Chesterton*, 1700).

Physiotherapy is considered to consist of three categories of treatment, known as 'the three pillars': manual therapy (hands-on techniques); electrotherapy (uses treatment machines); and exercise therapy (the use of exercise to treat, rather than for fitness). It is this last area which has much overlap with other professions, including that of therapists, trainers and fitness coaches.

That is where this book comes in. *The Complete Guide to Exercise Therapy* is a detailed examination of the importance of prescribing exercise therapy as rehabilitation to those who have been injured or for the prevention and management of pain. It is designed to give professionals administering exercise therapy everything they need to do it correctly and safely.

We begin with a presentation of the various body tissues, including muscles, ligaments, tendons and bone; how they heal and their reaction to both injury and rehabilitation. We investigate the healing timescale and establish a base upon which to competently assess injury before progressing the correct exercise techniques for successful treatment.

We then cover the essential foundations of exercise knowledge, including the importance of overload, adaptability and individuality, each of which feeds into pacing exercise progression

to the changes presenting in your client's body.

However, it is not just the choice of exercise which is important when providing your client with an effective treatment programme, but the way in which it is taught. Therefore, Chapter 5 assesses the methods for structuring a rehabilitation programme, including how to take into account your client's stamina, strength and stability, but also the psychological impact that an injury can have on day-to-day movement and activities. Chapter 6 then goes on to describe effective teaching methods, providing you with the tools and techniques to monitor and measure pain and tissue reaction to rehabilitation and encourage your client to progress through their treatment programme with appropriate goal-setting and feedback.

Finally, the second half of the book, specifically Chapters 7 to 14, provides you with a handbook of over a hundred exercise methods for the entire body, divided into the regions of: hip and thigh; knee; shin, ankle and foot; shoulder; elbow, wrist and hand; low back and pelvis; thoracic spine and chest; and head and neck. Each exercise includes detailed instructions and full-colour photo demonstrations to ensure you are exercising your client in the safest and most effective way. Clinical scenarios are also provided for common injuries, which illustrate how to form individual exercises into an effective and coherent programme. It is hoped that the comprehensive nature of the book means *The Complete Guide to Exercise Therapy* will become an essential tool for anyone administering exercise therapy in the treatment environment.

# HOW TISSUES HEAL

1

When you are managing injuries, it is essential to understand the process your client's tissues go through when they heal so you can work with their body's healing rather than against it. As healing progresses, your exercise therapy changes or progresses, so knowledge of the healing time-scale is vital.

## TYPES OF HEALING

The instigation of healing in damaged tissues depends on the proximity of the ends of the torn tissue filaments (stumps). Where the tissue stumps are close together in a minor injury (or following a surgical incision) a bridge is formed across the healing tissues and healing is said to be *primary* (known as 'healing by primary intension'). Where the tissues stumps have been pulled apart, a larger gap is formed between the injured tissue and *secondary* healing occurs. Now, new tissue is produced from the bottom and sides of the wound to gradually fill it and form a tissue plug rather than a bridge. In each case, healing progresses in distinct stages.

## INJURY AND INFLAMMATION

For convenience, the healing process can be divided into four interrelating phases (*see* Figure 1.1), and our exercise therapy prescription must match these phases. The first phase is injury itself, and already healing has started.

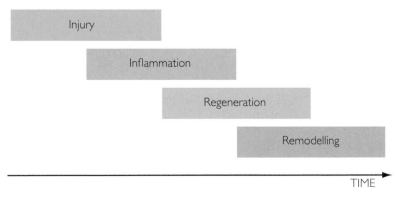

**Figure 1.1** The four phases of healing

## Injury

When soft tissue, such as muscle or ligament, is damaged some of the local blood capillaries running through it are disrupted, releasing fresh blood into the area. This has two important effects. First, as you will see below, the tissue disruption instigates chemical messages, which begin the healing process. Second, because the blood vessels are damaged fresh blood can no longer flow into the local tissues. Starved of new blood, which should bring with it oxygen and tissue nutrients, the tissues begin to die (a process known as *necrosis*). Think of this like watering your garden. If you cut the hosepipe, water doesn't get to the flowers and they dry up and die. The same is true here, except a blood vessel has been cut and the tissue rather than the flowers may wither. If you continue to exercise, the metabolic rate or 'tick over' of the tissues remains high and the demand for oxygen is increased. This increased demand speeds up tissue death, which occurs due to the oxygen shortage. Rest is therefore vital to slow the metabolic rate and reduce the oxygen demand. Exercise has a vital part to play later on in the healing process, but at this stage it is contraindicated. Instead, basic sports first aid is required.

> ### Definition
>
> Metabolic rate is the chemical 'tick over' of the body. It is the amount of oxygen and nutrients that your body requires just to keep going. Exercise increases metabolic rate while rest reduces it, much like putting your foot on a car accelerator pedal to use more petrol, and taking it off to use less.

Local cell death occurring in the injured tissues releases enzymes which begin the process of digesting and dissolving dead material. The body acts quickly as a natural 'road sweeper' to clean up the area in preparation for new tissue growth. This activity further stimulates the release of important chemicals, including *histamine* and *prostaglandin*, which act as chemical messengers.

As blood is released by damaged blood vessels, red blood cells are exposed to proteins, causing blood clotting to begin. The blood chemical *fibrin* beings to form a meshwork around the injured area, which then develops into a clot. The blood clot (haematoma) is an essential precursor to form a bridge between the ends of the torn tissue, and any movement which disrupts the clot slows the normal healing process. Continuing to exercise in the immediate post-injury phase is therefore detrimental.

> ### Keypoint
>
> Immediately after injury your tissues are disrupted and their blood flow reduced. Starved of new blood, tissue death occurs. Rest is vital to slow this process down.

## Inflammation

Inflammation begins 10 minutes after an injury occurs and may last several days depending on which sports first aid action you take. Inflammation gives four outward signs: *pain*; *heat*; *redness* and *swelling* (*see* Figure 1.2).

Heat and redness occur due to the increase in local blood flow, that is blood which flows close to the injured area. The increase develops as a result of blood vessels opening. Just as your

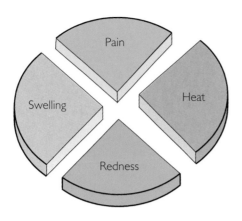

**Figure 1.2** The four outward signs of inflammation

skin becomes red as your body heats up during exercise, the local skin surrounding an injury reddens. However, this will only be noticeable where the damaged tissues are close to the surface (also known as 'superficial'). When you sprain your ankle, the area feels hot and looks red, but if you damage your back, where the damaged tissues lie much deeper, the area may feel hot to you but to an outside observer redness is rarely noticeable unless the condition is very severe. Again the process is brought about by a number of chemicals including prostaglandin, and it is this chemical that non-steroidal anti-inflammatory drugs (NSAIDs) work on to calm the inflammation.

**Definition**

Non-steroidal anti-inflammatory drugs (e.g. ibuprofen) are used to reduce pain and inflammation, especially in joint and muscle conditions.

The broken blood vessels cause blood flow to slow. The blood cells themselves become sticky, adhering to the vessel walls to form part of the developing blood clot which dams the area to stop further bleeding into the damaged tissues.

### Swelling

*Swelling* (also called 'oedema') begins as the slow blood movement is unable to keep pace with the fluids being formed by the body. As the damaged tissues release their chemicals, the body tries to dilute the area with watery fluid, which is the basis of swelling. The swelling moves into the lymphatic vessels and should be taken away as part of the normal lymph flow process.

**Definition**

The lymphatic system is part of the circulatory system. Its network of fine tubes exists in addition to the blood vessels, carrying a clear fluid called 'lymph'. Blood does not directly contact tissues, rather blood cells remain in the vessels while lymph seeps out to touch the tissues directly.

Unfortunately, the sheer volume of swelling that often develops after a sports injury means some of the watery fluid settles and pools around the injured area. Initially the swelling is a watery fluid, but it contains similar clotting chemicals to blood, which over time becomes firmer and gel-like. If left, over many weeks the gel-like swelling can harden still further. One of the aims of an exercise therapist should be to restrict the spread of this sticky swelling so it affects a smaller area. This is one function of elastic supports and taping. Another useful tool is massage, which aims to remove excess swelling and stave off the problem of the tissue becoming stuck together (also known as 'consolidated oedema').

### Keypoint

Following injury you must aim to stem the spread of swelling.

## Pain

Pain is an inevitable consequence of sports injuries, and occurs because the chemicals produced at the time of injury irritate the nerve sensors within the tissues. As swelling occurs, the pressure of the developing fluids presses on the sensors and further pain is produced.

Pain is created by tiny electrical nervous impulses travelling from the tissue sensors to the brain. This feeling (sensory) mechanism consists of nerves which travel as a *pain pathway*, first to the spinal cord. Here they form a junction (synapse) with a small intermediate nerve (interneuron), which itself connects to a longer fibre travelling to the brain where the pain is actually felt. Even within the brain there are several nerve connections (*see* Figure 1.3). At each junction between the nerves, the nervous impulse can be changed. This fact is important both for pain relief and for the development of longer term (chronic) pain. If another nerve impulse arrives at the nerve junction in the spine, it can cancel out the painful signal. This is what happens when you knock your knee and 'rub it better'. The vigorous rubbing causes an intense

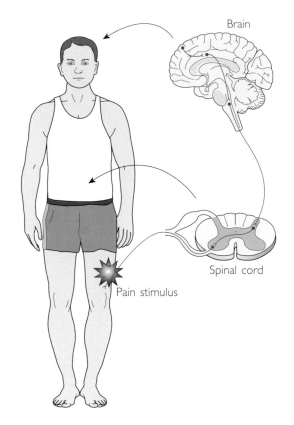

**Figure 1.3** Nerve connections within the brain

sensory stimulus which cancels out the pain at the level of the spinal cord, an effect called 'counterirritation'.

As the nerve impulse travels into the brain, you feel pain (known as 'sensory perception'). However, the impulse also travels across junctions

### Definition

A counterirritant effect is caused when a second intense stimulus cancels out a painful feeling. The effect occurs at the junction between two sensory nerves.

to other nerves going to different brain areas. Some go to emotional centres, and so intense pain – especially if it occurs over a prolonged period – can cause emotional changes, such as fear of movement. Fear of this type is important to consider when prescribing exercise therapy following a severe injury, such as a broken leg or car accident for example, when exercise therapy is vital for full recovery. Without it, the client may be pain free but will never have full function of the injured body part.

The nerve junctions can also work to the therapist's advantage. You can reduce or block pain using treatments such as heat, massage and ice. Impulses produced by the brain as a result of these treatments can flood the body with pain-relieving chemicals and also remove the fear of movement. This type of pain relief is called 'descending inhibition' and it is caused by many common treatments, such as heat and ice. Both descending inhibition and the reduction of fear of movement are known to occur when using exercise. In fact, the use of graded exercise programmes for patients suffering with chronic pain, for example, are now at the forefront of pain research.

## Keypoint

Graded exercise therapy (GET), physical activity that starts slowly and gradually increases throughout the treatment process, is commonly used as part of the management of chronic pain.

# THE HEALING TIMESCALE

The process of tissue healing can take some time. Minor knocks may resolve in a matter of days while major injuries can take many months and sometimes even years to heal completely. The key to the healing timescale is the amount of tissue damage you have, and how the injury is treated. The process of healing described above proceeds through three interrelated phases: *acute*, *subacute* and *chronic*.

## ACUTE PHASE

During the *acute phase* your tissues have been damaged and are reacting to this. It is the stage of *inflammation* (*see* page 8). There is local bleeding and swelling. Your tissues have not yet started to heal and so your aim should be damage limitation – you must not take any action which stresses the damaged tissues and further injures them. Trying to run off an injury or play with painkillers blocking out the pain can induce more tissue damage than actually occurred in the initial injury. In addition, we have seen that the swelling formed at the time of injury can spread throughout the local area. Limiting this spread is vital because the sticky swelling clots, and if it travels further, it affects more tissue. The acute phase of healing typically lasts 48 hours and ceases when the tissues begin to form a healing bridge across the damaged area.

## SUBACUTE PHASE

When the healing tissues start to form and no fresh swelling or bleeding occurs, you have entered the *subacute phase* of healing, which may last anything from 14 to 21 days. This is the stage of *regeneration*, when tissue regrowth begins. Initially a soft blood clot forms and a stronger tissue mesh begins to grow around the area. The new healing tissue forms a scar in the same way the skin heals after a cut. This tissue shrinks and pulls its torn ends together, effectively bridging the tissue gap. The tissue formed at this stage of healing has fibres which are arranged in a haphazard (known as 'disorganised') fashion. The finished tissue must have fibres which align in the strongest direction possible (known as 'organised' – *see* 'Scar tissue' below for further information).

### Chronic phase

The final stage of the healing timescale is the *chronic phase*, which is the stage of *remodelling* lasting from 21 days onwards. Although the term 'chronic' is used here, this phase is an essential stage in which your scar tissue adapts to become more like the original tissue it has replaced. Exercise is vital during this stage, and if it is too gentle, the tissue will not be stressed sufficiently to adapt fully. The tissue stress shouldn't just be intense, but must closely match that which occurs in sport. In other words, the stresses imposed on the healed tissue must be *functional* (*see* Chapter 3 for further information).

The remodelling phase can last for many years, and one of the mistakes which is often made during rehabilitation is to stop too soon. Although your tissue may be relatively pain free when healed by 80 per cent, it is still not fully functional. In other words, when subjected to the severe stress of competitive sport your tissue may fail. During this phase it is vital that a sportsperson has a graded rehabilitation programme which lasts long enough – at least 3–4 months. Many of us find this odd and think 'Surely my injury will not last that long?', but this misses an essential feature of healing, which

is *tissue adaptation*. If you join a gym and begin performing a bench press, you should expect to improve the weight you are able to lift over a period of time. The improvement is a result of tissue adaptation, with the chest and arm muscles (pectorals and triceps) getting stronger. You would not just give up in a matter of weeks, but would continue with your programme over months and years. Why? Because you know the muscles will continue to strengthen, providing your training is correct. The same is true of tissue adaptation following injury. If the rehab program is correct, tissue adaptation continues for many months.

## SCAR TISSUE

We have seen that as healing progresses new tissue is formed. This tissue is a meshwork of fibres formed from fibrous tissue. Fibrous tissue contains two main types of fibres, one which is strong (fibrin), the other more elastic (elastin). The amount of each of these fibres is governed by the requirements of the tissue. For example, both tendons at the ends of muscles and ligaments supporting joints are made of fibrous tissue. However, ligaments are more stretchy than tendons and so have a greater proportion of elastin fibres than fibrin. As your injury heals, it is vital that your tissue remodels to closely resemble the original tissue format. If it is too loose or too tight, its function will be impaired. The make-up of fibrous tissue changes depending on the stress placed upon it.

We have seen that after injury a blood clot forms (*see* Figure 1.4a) and shrinks (*see* Figure 1.4b). The healing meshwork of fibrous tissue begins to form and has a haphazard appearance,

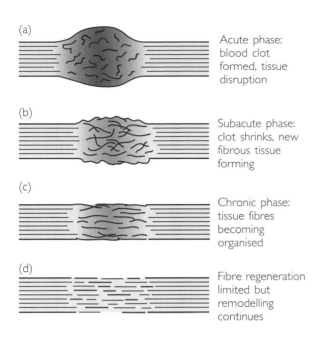

(a) Acute phase: blood clot formed, tissue disruption

(b) Subacute phase: clot shrinks, new fibrous tissue forming

(c) Chronic phase: tissue fibres becoming organised

(d) Fibre regeneration limited but remodelling continues

**Figure 1.4** After injury, a blood clot forms (a) and shrinks (b). The tissues form in a disorganised fashion (c) and then start to align in an organised pattern (d).

with fibres pointing in various directions (*see* Figure 1.4c). The finished tissue must have fibres which align in the strongest direction possible (*see* Figure 1.4d) to take on the function of the original tissue.

To change from the haphazard fibre orientation to a more organised mesh, the tissue must be stressed slightly. As we have seen, too little stress and the fibres will not align correctly, but with too much stress the fibres break down again. Progressive exercise in the subacute phase is the key (*see* 'Graded exercise therapy', page 11).

# MUSCLE ADAPTATION TO INJURY AND DISUSE

One of the tissues most affected by injury is muscle. It becomes weaker and shrinks (wastes) due to pain. Muscle wastage occurs through changes in nervous impulses. Even at rest your muscles usually receive constant nerve impulses to keep them ready for action. It is this 'resting tone' which gives muscles their natural firmness. The tone reduces if the muscle is not used because fewer nervous impulses get through. The flabby muscle appearance is called 'disuse atrophy'.

When a joint swells and is painful, the body tries to protect itself by preventing movement. Now the muscle tone drops off very quickly (within 24 hours). In this case it is not just a reduction in nervous impulses which normally tell the muscle to stay firm, but an increase in other impulses which deliberately tell the muscle to relax, a condition called 'muscular inhibition'. Moving a painful joint increases these new nervous impulses and intensifies the muscular inhibition. Protecting a painful swollen joint from movement is therefore vital, and this is the job of taping and splinting. For further details see the *Complete Guide to Sports Injuries* (Norris, 2011), published by Bloomsbury.

Following injury it is vital that your muscle strength be increased to pre-injury levels. However, there are a number of considerations

> **Keypoint**
>
> *Disuse atrophy* is muscle wasting due to lack of use. *Muscle inhibition* is wasting due to nerve impulses created by pain and swelling.

to take before proceeding with treatment. First, muscle will not strengthen effectively where pain still exists. Strength training produces nerve signals telling a muscle to increase its tone, while pain produces other signals telling the muscle to reduce tone. The result is the two forms of stimuli cancel each other out and the muscle does not strengthen. Gentle exercise may be used when pain is present to increase the flow of fluids (blood and lymph) around the area, but pain should never increase. Once pain has subsided, gentle exercise may give way to strengthening (*see* Chapter 3).

The second consideration when using exercise is the presence of *movement dysfunction*. Here, the quality of a movement will have degraded due to pain. An everyday example of movement dysfunction is a limp. When you get a stone in your shoe, the pressure on the sole of your foot causes you to change the way you walk to avoid the pain. With each step you are in fact practising a new form of walking – literally rehearsing your limp. After some time, if you take the stone out of your shoe, you will still limp because you have now practised the movement dysfunction and it has become a habit. If you decide to use walking as part of a training programme, you further reinforce the movement dysfunction, and although you may walk faster because you have increased your movement quantity, the movement quality is poor. It is therefore vital to undo the limp (correct the movement dysfunction) before you increase the amount of exercise you do. One of the fundamental underpinnings of rehabilitation is to address movement quality before movement quantity.

### Keypoint

Correct movement quality (how an exercise is performed) before quantity (how many repetitions of an exercise you can do).

# TISSUE REACTION TO INJURY AND REHABILITATION

2

For accurate exercise therapy prescription we need to appreciate what happens to the tissues during injury, and how they change during rehabilitation. Our aim, of course, is to match one with the other, improving the tissue condition. Any mismatch between the stress imposed on the tissues through exercise and the ability of the tissues to adapt may interfere with the healing process or, worse still, result in an outright injury. Let's look at some of the tissues most commonly affected by injury (*see* Figure 2.1).

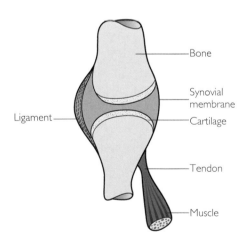

**Figure 2.1** Tissues affected by musculoskeletal (MSK) injury

## MUSCLE

### CHANGES DUE TO REHABILITATION

Muscle is an important tissue both for its reaction to injury and its ability to adapt by strengthening to support a joint. Two types of changes occur to muscle through training; one is *structural*, the other *functional*.

> **Keypoint**
>
> A *structural* change is an alteration in the physical make-up of tissue, while a *functional* change is an alteration in the way a tissue acts.

### Structural changes

Structural changes (called *myogenic*) involve an increase in the amount of muscle protein and the growth of blood vessels into the muscle to make its contraction more effective. Alteration of muscle protein causes the muscle to become larger or hypertrophy, with average values of 30 per cent greater muscle fibre diameter and 45 per cent more nuclei. Both slow twitch (type I) and fast twitch (type II) fibres may increase, with changes favouring one type over the other (known as 'selective hypertrophy') being dependent on training type. Although the total number of muscle fibres remains very much the same, endurance training favours slow twitch fibre hypertrophy while heavy resistance training encourages fast twitch (type II and IIA) hypertrophy. In parallel with changes in muscle fibre size, connective tissue proliferation is seen with thickening of the muscle-tendon connection occurring over time.

In addition there are changes to the chemicals of the muscle, making it better able to cope with the increased work of training. Endurance training especially increases the amount of energy-storing chemicals (adenosine triphosphate (ATP) and creatine phosphate (CP)) and the enzymes responsible for energy production within the muscle (phosphofructokinase and lactate dehydrogenase).

Changes of this type are typically thought to be the preserve of young healthy individuals. However, these same changes can be brought about in seniors as part of an active ageing programme. Research studies have shown increases in muscle volume (26 per cent) and work output (28 per cent) in men with an average age of 67. Studies have also shown increases in muscle cross-sectional area and functional strength, including during stair climbing tasks and gait velocity (Fiatrone 1994, Sipala and Suominen 1995).

## Functional changes

Structural changes do not occur immediately when you start training. In fact, long before, there are functional changes (*neurogenic*) which make the muscles work more smoothly and effectively, demonstrated by increased electromyography (EMG) activity. Motor units within the muscle increase their firing rate (frequency) and the

> ### Definition
>
> A *motor unit* consists of a single nerve fibre (a motor neuron) and the muscle fibres it supplies. The number of motor units per muscle varies with large muscles, such as quadriceps, having about 1000 and small muscles, such as those in the eye, having perhaps 10.

number of motor units used increases (volume). In addition the motor units contract together in a more coordinated fashion (known as 'motor unit synchronisation').

With ageing, the size and strength of a muscle reduces, a process called *sarcopenia*, and this characteristic has important implications for exercise therapy with seniors. Sarcopenia sees a reduction in the size of all types of muscle fibres, with type II fibre size reduction occurring more rapidly than type I. Reduction in muscle mass (circumference) and gait impairment (walking speed) are typically used as diagnostic indicators. In addition to changes in fibre circumference there is an increase of both connective tissue within the muscle (known as 'fibrosis') and fat infiltration.

Functional changes involve the electrical charges travelling through the nerve and muscle and the coordination between the muscle fibres, making them contract together as a team rather than in a haphazard fashion. In addition, when you first start training, your body will not allow you to contract your muscles maximally. It does this because the pain of lifting weights is identified as a potential threat that could injure the muscle. Your body stops you contracting your muscles maximally by preventing the nervous impulses getting through to the muscle (a process called *inhibition*). As you train, you begin to realise the aching and soreness you get is very different from the pain of injury, and your body begins to allow you to work your muscles harder by removing the inhibition on the muscle (known as *disinhibition*).

## CHANGES DUE TO INJURY

Injury to muscle may be either *direct* or *indirect*. Direct injury is through a blow, such as a knee striking an opponent's body in rugby. A direct blow causes a compressive force leading to muscle contusion (bruising) while force over a more confined area (a boot stud, for example) causes laceration (cutting or splitting) to the skin initially or unusually to the muscle itself. Indirect injury causes muscle strain, normally to biarticular (two-joint) muscles such as the hamstrings, rectus femoris and gastrocnemius of the lower limb or biceps or triceps of the upper limb. The coordination of a biarticular muscle is more complex than that of a uniarticular (single-joint) muscle and injury typically occurs during rapid acceleration or deceleration, especially when an athlete is fatigued.

The contractile elements of the muscle are injured in the first instance, typically at the musculotendinous junction where force is applied.

Greater force may cause a mid-belly tear and even greater force damage to the connective tissue framework of the muscle (cytoskeleton).

Muscle heals by *repair* while bone heals by *regeneration*. The essential difference is repair involves the formation of a healing bridge (or scar, *see* page 12) while bone regenerates so that the new tissue will eventually be identical to the damaged area (*see* below).

### Keypoint

*Repair* causes replacement tissue by formation of a scar. *Regeneration* is by formation of new material, which is identical to the damaged tissue.

We saw in Chapter 1 how soft tissues heal, and with muscle a similar process occurs (*see* Table 2.1). The myofibrils or contractile element of the muscle (containing actin and myosin molecules) have been torn apart through injury and the dead material is removed by scavenging white blood cells (macrophages), in a process known as 'phagocytosis'. Scar tissue is formed across

| Table 2.1 | The phases of muscle healing | |
|---|---|---|
| **Destruction** | **Repair** | **Remodelling** |
| • Rupture of myofibres | • Phagocytosis of necrotic tissue | • Maturation of regenerated myofibres |
| • Tissue necrosis | • Regeneration of myofibres | |
| • Haematoma between myofibre stumps | • Connective tissue scar formed | • Retraction and reorganisation of scar |
| • Inflammatory reaction | • Revascularisation and ingrowth of capillaries | • Recovery of functional capacity of muscle |

Data from Jarvinen *et al* 2007

this dead region and dormant satellite cells at the end of the muscle become activated as part of the repair process. Regenerating muscle cells reach out across the dead zone of the injured muscle and press through the scar. In turn the scar shrinks and the regenerating muscle fibres from each side fuse. Eventually the muscle returns to full function with little scar tissue remaining.

# BONE

Clients with a bony injury normally require rehabilitation after the bone break has healed, so a basic knowledge of fractures and healing is required by all exercise professionals prescribing rehab.

## BONE MAKE-UP

Bone types are classified according to their shape. Four types are typically described:
1. Long (in the limbs)
2. Short (at the ankles and wrists)
3. Flat (scapula and pelvis)
4. Irregular (vertebrae).

Each is made up of two different types of bone: *cancellous* (also called 'spongy') and *compact*.

Cancellous bone consists of a network of fine struts called *trabeculae* which are aligned in the direction of imposed force upon the bone (*see* Figure 2.2).

Some stress on bone is therefore essential, otherwise the trabeculae will be haphazard in alignment, making the bone weaker.

Compact bone forms the shaft of long bones, such as the femur (thighbone) and humerus (upper arm bone), and the centre is hollow (known as a 'medullary cavity') and filled with bone marrow.

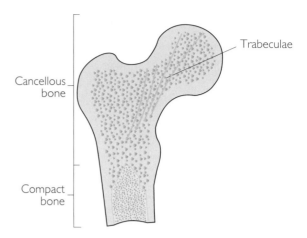

**Figure 2.2** Cancellous and compact bone

The marrow is red in children, but in adults only around half is red, the rest being yellow. Red marrow is responsible for the production of red blood cells (used to carry oxygen), white blood cells (used for immunity) and platelets (used for blood clotting). Yellow marrow consists mainly of fat, but the body has the ability to convert the yellow marrow back into red in cases of blood loss. Both types contain stem cells (*mesenchymal stem cells*) which are capable of developing into other tissue cells, and these may be taken medically (harvested) from the bone forming the crest of the pelvis (iliac crest).

Bone combines elasticity and rigidity because it consists of a matrix impregnated with calcium salts. The calcium salts form a ready store of calcium for body processes and can be moved into and out of the body fluids. The rate at which this happens depends on a number of factors, including loading through activity and exercise and hormonal influences. Where a client has osteoporosis, calcium salts are leeched from the bone making them weaker (known as 'rarefied'). Treatment of this condition involves a combination of diet to ensure sufficient calcium is taken, hormonal medication and exercise to slow the process at which calcium is taken from the bone.

Bone is encased by a thin membrane, the periosteum, which is highly vascular. The deep surface of this membrane which is closest to the bone contains bone-forming cells known as *osteoblasts*. A direct blow to the bone (from a hockey ball on the unprotected shin, for example) can cause bruising between the periosteum and bone which lifts the membrane away from the bone. The ensuing gap is filled with bone salts giving a permanent lump, the reason it is vital to encourage young sportsmen and women to wear shin pads when playing football or hockey.

## BONE GROWTH AND DEVELOPMENT

Bone begins to form when the child is still in the womb (7–12 weeks intrauterine) and begins as cartilage. Bone growth and development (*see* Figure 2.3) starts with bone formation (ossification) in the shaft and spreads outwards from this central point which is known as the 'primary ossification centre' or 'diaphysis'. Secondary ossification centres

(epiphyses) appear at the bone ends and the two centres expand towards each other until only a thin layer of cartilage separates them. This thin layer is called the growth plate (epiphyseal plate) and is where the bone continues to lengthen during the adolescent growth spur. If it is damaged by a fracture, bone growth may be impaired.

### Keypoint

Damage to the bone growth plate can be very serious and where it is suspected, referral for X-ray or scan is imperative.

## TREATING BONE DAMAGE

Damage to the growth plate can be of various types:

- *Shearing stress* can cause the bone end to slip relative to the bone shaft. Compressing can close the growth plate, preventing further bone growth. A fracture of the bone end can cause the growth plate to split.

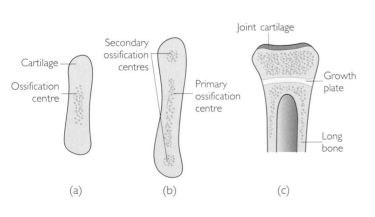

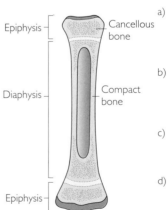

a) Cartilage model of bone during foetal life with ossification centre established

b) Development of primary and secondary ossification centres in early life

c) Growth plate (epiphyseal plate) during adolescence

d) Adult bone showing division into compact bone shaft (diaphysis) and cancellous bone ends (epiphyses)

**Figure 2.3** The stages of bone growth and development

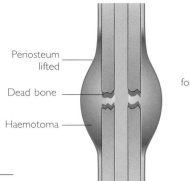
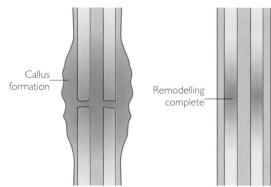

Periosteum lifted

Dead bone

Haemotoma

Callus formation

Remodelling complete

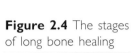

**Figure 2.4** The stages of long bone healing

Fractures to bone may be either traumatic through sudden injury (bone break) or gradual onset through overuse (stress fracture). Healing of a long bone progresses in a number of stages (*see* Figure 2.4). Initially local blood vessels are torn and a blood clot is formed. The escaping blood is contained by the periosteum, and the area of bone close to the damaged site begins to die back. Bone cells begin to be formed from the underside of the periosteum and the damaged medullary cavity, and new blood capillaries form. Bone cell activity increases with new bone formed and dead bone debris removed, with new bone visable on an X-ray as callus. New bone is gradually remodelled and reshaped to match the pre-injured site. The total healing process varies depending on the site of injury with callus visible on an X-ray by 2–3 weeks, and full healing taking from 8–16 weeks. Cancellous bone heals more quickly because it does not contact a medullary cavity and so the contact area between the two sides of the fracture site is greater.

## OSTEOARTHROSIS

Both bone and hyaline cartilage are involved in osteoarthritis (sometimes called osteoarthrosis or simply OA), and this responds well to exercise therapy, so let's take a look at the condition.

The initial change is to the hyaline cartilage at the ends of the bone. The water content of the cartilage increases due to chemical changes and the surface of the cartilage begins to fray. This is most noticeable in the areas at the side of the joint which are not weight bearing. Later, damage occurs to the deeper layers of the cartilage in a process called 'fibrillation'. The cartilage begins to blister and small pieces may detach and float within the joint fluid (synovial fluid) as so-called loose bodies, causing clicking and twinges of pain. The cartilage begins to thin, reducing the distance between the bones, and on X-ray the appearance is of a reduced joint space. The bone directly beneath the cartilage (subchondral bone) becomes smooth and shiny in a process called 'eburnation'. The synovial membrane of the joint becomes thicker and less elastic, stiffening the joint, and the joint capsule can develop small tears which repair with scar tissue, reducing the elasticity or springiness of the joint.

### Keypoint

In OA, joint cartilage suffers *fibrillation*, becoming flaky, and the bone beneath suffers *eburnation*, becoming smooth and shiny. Soft tissues around the joint stiffen.

## LIGAMENTS

Ligaments are tough bands consisting of collagen fibres. Articular ligaments are the most common type and these join bone to bone (*see* Figure 2.5). They may be positioned outside the joint (extracapsular) where they reinforce the joint capsule (for example, the medial collateral ligament of the knee) or within the joint (intracapsular) where they act directly on the bone (for example, the anterior cruciate ligament of the knee).

> ### Keypoint
>
> An *extracapsular* ligament lies on the surface of a joint, while an *intracapsular* ligament lies within the joint.

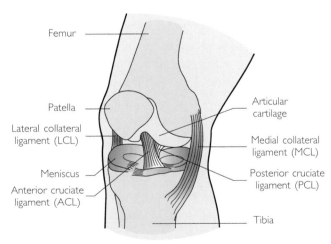

Femur

Patella

Lateral collateral
ligament (LCL)

Meniscus

Anterior cruciate
ligament (ACL)

Articular
cartilage

Medial collateral
ligament (MCL)

Posterior cruciate
ligament (PCL)

Tibia

**Figure 2.5** Articular ligaments join bone to bone

## LIGAMENT MAKE-UP

Ligament fibres are arranged in lines (linearly) which fan out as the ligament attaches to bone to spread the load more evenly. Each ligament fibre has a wavy or 'crimped' appearance under a microscope, and as the ligament is stretched the crimps straighten out, tightening the ligament. The crimps actually give the ligament its elasticity (pseudoelasticity) because the ligament itself contains little elastic material. In fact, most ligaments contain no more than 1–2 degrees of elastic fibres (type I collagen).

The crimps and fanning out of the ligament at its attachment also give the ligament another feature: as it is placed on stretch it actually becomes stronger. This is because the fibres stretch out and take up slack so that they align in the direction of the imposed force. This is important for rehabilitation because this process can be reduced by the formation of scar tissue after injury, and depends on movement for its restoration.

## LIGAMENT DAMAGE

Ligaments display a feature called viscoelasticity. They are stretchy and give joints a healthy springy feeling when stretched initially, but if the stretch is continued for a prolonged period, the ligament gradually gives and the tissue then becomes weaker. We call this feature *hysteresis*, and it is important to injury. Take as an example someone who bends forwards. They stretch their spinal ligaments and as they stand up the ligaments recoil back to their original shape. However, if this person bends over for a prolonged period, for example, if they are working at a bench, the ligaments are placed on stretch and held in that position. They gradually pay out and when the person eventually straightens up the ligaments remain lengthened (and slightly weaker) for some time. In some cases it can take 1–2 hours for ligaments to return to their pre-stretched state, leaving the joint less stable and susceptible to injury during that time.

Ligaments contain small sensory nerve endings, some relaying feelings of discomfort (pain receptors) and others giving information about tension (mechanoreceptors). After an injury where pain and swelling has occurred, the mechanoreceptors can be damaged and this gives rise to a reduction in joint position sense (or 'proprioception'), making the joint less stable and creating a tendency for it to give way. Proprioceptive training is therefore an important part of the rehabilitation process following a joint injury.

## Keypoint

Damage to mechanoreceptors in ligaments can impair joint position sense following injury. Proprioceptive training as part of the rehabilitation process can help restore this.

# SYNOVIAL MEMBRANE AND FLUID

Synovial membrane lines fluid-filled (synovial) joints. The membrane has two layers and contains cells (synoviocytes) which produce a substance called hyaluronate (or hyaluronic acid) which acts as a lubricant. Synovial membrane is highly vascular and has numerous folds which open up like a bellows as the joint bends and straightens. If the joint swells, the folds in the synovium are placed under stretch and the joint will not move as easily, contributing to joint stiffness.

The amount of synovial fluid contained within a joint may be very little (2–4ml) and this is spread throughout the joint, with some of it being stored in fat pads and pouches (known as 'bursa') around the joint. The fluid is thick and syrupy (or viscous) and with movement it becomes thinner and more mobile, making the joint less stiff. As the joint moves the fluid is sloshed across the joint surface bringing nutrients to the joint cartilage, and as the joint takes weight some of the nutrient substances are pressed into the cartilage. Continued movement is therefore essential for joint health.

## SYNOVIAL MEMBRANE DAMAGE

With a minor injury the synovial membrane is not structurally damaged, but its blood vessels open (known as a 'vasomotor reaction'), its metabolic rate increases and more joint fluid is produced. This process causes minor joint swelling and is known as a *traumatic synovitis*. If the process continues, the synovial membrane thickens and releases protein cells into the joint fluid causing self-perpetuation of the swelling, giving a *reactive synovitis*. The joint will be swollen, hot and painful and the reaction occurs quite slowly after injury (within 12–24 hours), with the effects possibly lasting for up to 3 weeks. Where immediate swelling occurs (within 1–2 hours after injury) and pain is more intense, the indication is of *haemarthrosis* or blood in the joint from a more major injury which has torn blood vessels rather than just opened them up.

# TENDONS

Tendons join muscles to bone and as such transmit high forces onto fairly small contact areas. They must be both firm enough to transmit force, but elastic enough to allow movement when a joint is bending and straightening. Although tendons transmit force produced by the muscle rather than create it themselves, they can store force and then release it. This is because of their elastic nature, so, for example, during running the Achilles tendon is stretched much like an elastic band as you close your ankle joint (dorsiflex). The recoil from this action is released as you move forwards as a force to point your toes (plantarflex). In this way force from motion is reused, reducing the requirement on muscle to create all of the force for the running action. Forces in running have been calculated to be over eight times a person's bodyweight with every step, so the Achilles tendon is a truly remarkable structure to be able to withstand this day in and day out. The elasticity of the tendon also acts as a damper as well. If you jump down from a height, the force transmitted to your knee, hip and spine is reduced (damped) by the stretch of your Achilles tendon, which slows and absorbs (attenuates) the sudden shockwave of force that would be transmitted up the leg bones.

## TENDON MAKE-UP

Tendons consist of connective tissue (collagen) bundles grouped together. Each group is surrounded by a membrane (endotendon) and the various groups are surrounded by a final membrane called the epitendon and finally surrounded by a fairly loose sheet called the paratendon, which is lined by synovial cells to augment gliding. Some tendons glide even more freely because they have a double walled tendon sheath, which in the case of the tendons at the wrist or foot may have a number of tendons running within it.

## TENDON DAMAGE

We are all familiar with the way muscles change with training, becoming stronger and larger. However, what people often do not realise is tendons also change with training. They are dynamic (capable of responding and adapting) and metabolically active, with substances moving into and out of the tendon tissue regularly.

Tendons react to injury in a variety of ways and the generic term for the group of conditions giving pain in tendons is *tendinopathy*:

- *Tendonitis* is inflammation (swelling) of the tendon.
- *Paratendonitis* or *tenosynovitis* is inflammation of the tendon sheath.
- *Tenovaginitis* is roughening of the inner aspect of the sheath giving a grating (crepitus) sensation.
- *Tendinosis* is mild degeneration of the tendon substance and ruptures (tearing) may occur through either part of the tendon (partial rupture) or the whole tendon (complete rupture).

Overuse injury causes tendons to inflame for the short term, but over the long term the tendon tissue begins to react to the stress by thickening. In fact, a client with tendinopathy of the Achilles may show the tendon to double in thickness compared to the unaffected side. The collagen fibres within the tendon separate and degrade and the gap between them fills with a jelly-like connective tissue material (known as 'ground substance'). These changes cause the tendon to become less elastic and open to further injury. The tendon cells become more active and new blood vessels grow into the tendon (known as 'increased vascularity'), often dragging small nerve fibres in with them, which causes dull aching and pain on movement.

The fact that a tendon changes (adapts) as a result of stress is one of the keys to treatment because exercise therapy can cause the injured

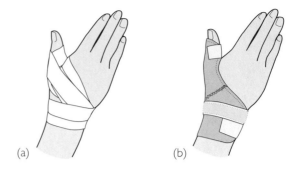

(a)          (b)

**Figure 2.6** Supporting a painful tendon

tendon to heal properly. The exercise must match the healing of the tendon, however, because too much increases tissue damage and too little will not load the tendon sufficiently to stimulate the tendon tissue to change. Initially, rest may be called for, with taping or splinting to protect the tendon from excessive force (*see* Figure 2.6). As pain resolves exercise therapy can begin.

# FOUNDATIONS OF EXERCISE KNOWLEDGE

# 3

When you exercise, your body changes in two important ways. The first is immediate and is called the exercise *response*. Your heart and breathing rate increase. You get warm and begin to sweat. Your muscles fill with blood and they use energy and produce waste products, which cause them to ache. When you stop exercising these processes gradually slow down and your body returns to normal. If you repeat the exercise bout, the same changes occur, but over a period of time your body becomes better at coping with the exercise. You sweat less, your heart and breathing rate are not as high, and you can exercise for longer periods before you ache. The longer term changes represent exercise *adaptation*.

## OVERLOAD AND ADAPTATION

Exercise must challenge the body tissues to be effective, and this challenge is called *overload*. When the body is overloaded, tissue breaks down at a microscopic level and rebuilds itself to become stronger, a process called *supercompensation*. To achieve this, exercise must challenge the body to a greater extent than normal day-to-day activities. For example, if we perform an arm curl exercise, the action (elbow flexion) is similar to picking up a teacup. We would not expect to strengthen the arm bending muscle (the biceps) by picking up a teacup because although the action is the same, the overload is not great enough.

## THE GENERAL ADAPTION SYNDROME (GAS)

Adaptation to exercise (a physical stress) can be understood through the principles of the General Adaptation Syndrome (GAS), first described by the Hungarian endocrinologist Hans Selye in the 1930s with reference to psychological stress. Plotting time against resistance to stress (*see* Figure 3.1a), the GAS consists of three phases. The first is the *alarm* phase as the body reacts by preparing its 'fight or flight' mechanisms releasing hormones such as adrenalin and cortisol. Phase two is the *resistance* phase when the body tries to cope with the imposed stress. The final phase is *exhaustion* when the body has depleted its coping mechanisms and may suffer from pathologies such as high blood pressure or ulcers, for example. The key to the GAS is the body can either positively adapt (called *eustress*), such as when it becomes stronger through weight training, or negatively adapt (called *distress*), for example, by overtraining.

(a) General Adaption Syndrome (GAS)

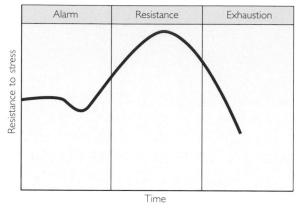

(b) Supercompensation

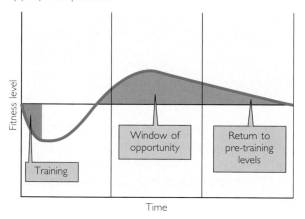

**Figure 3.1** The General Adaptation Syndrome (GAS)

The GAS is modified slightly when the imposed stress is exercise. The initial physical stress (exercise) is an overload which is at a higher level than that normally encountered. This stress causes body reactions which are physiological, biomechanical and psychological in nature. Immediately after training, fatigue in all three areas causes the body to be less able to react to an imposed stressor. For example, following heavy weight training, muscles feel exhausted and the mind lacks motivation (*see* Figure 3.1b). The

body gradually recovers, a process which may take 1 or 2 days and even up to a week if the imposed stress is very great (running a marathon, for example). As the body adapts, pre-exercise levels are restored, but the adaptation continues (known as 'supercompensation') so that the body become better equipped to cope with imposed stress. During this period further exercise causes the whole cycle to be repeated, but this time as the starting point (fitness level) is higher, the compensation is greater. For this reason the period of supercompensation is often referred to as the *window of opportunity*. Two key points emerge from this process. The first is that the body has to be given the opportunity to adapt with adequate rest and good nutrition, for example. The second is that the next training period must occur during the window of opportunity. Clearly if the next training period occurs too soon the body won't have finished adapting, but if it occurs too late, the body will have returned to pre-training fitness levels.

## Keypoint

Following training, the body must be given time to recover for maximal tissue adaptation to occur.

The overload is made up of four factors described by the simple pneumonic FITT, which stands for *frequency*, *intensity*, *time* and *type*:

- *Frequency* is how often you practise an exercise, for example, twice a day or three times a week.
- *Intensity* describes how hard an exercise is. In

strength training, this is normally measured in comparison to the maximum weight you can lift once (1 repetition maximum or 1RM) or the maximum voluntary contraction (MVC) of a muscle. With stretching it is how far you stretch as a proportion to your maximum range of movement (ROM), for example, 60% max ROM or 80% max ROM.

- *Time* is the duration of the exercise, for example, running for 20 minutes or 1 hour. It also refers to the duration of a repetition, for example, using a very slow action (known as 'superslow technique') in weight training to emphasise muscle contraction.

- *Type* is the category of exercise, such as strength training, aerobics, stretching, plyometrics, and each of these can be subdivided depending on which of the 'S' factors of fitness are worked (see below).

These four factors are called *training variables* (*see* Table 3.1), and altering any of them changes the overall work intensity. The total amount of work is often expressed in sets and reps, and together the description of an exercise using these variables is commonly referred to as *training volume*.

| Table 3.1 | Training variables |
|-----------|--------------------|
| **Variable** | **Meaning** |
| Type | Exercise category (weight training, stretching, etc.) |
| Duration | How long exercise lasts |
| Frequency | How often exercise is practised (daily, weekly, etc.) |
| Intensity | How hard exercise is |

> ### Keypoint
>
> *Training volume* is the total amount of work performed during an exercise by combining the training variables of frequency, intensity, time and type.

For example, heavy weight training is clearly harder than light jogging (exercise type), while slow walking is easier than fast walking (intensity). Performing a trunk curl exercise every hour throughout the day is harder than performing it every other day (frequency) and performing 10 reps is easier than 100 reps (duration). Performing the trunk curl everyday for 3 sets of 10 reps gives a larger training volume than performing it three times each week for 2 sets of 12 reps.

## REVERSIBILITY

Failure to overload tissue sufficiently (*detraining*) results in loss of the benefits gained as part of the training adaptation. This loss is termed *reversibility* and equates to the simple adage 'use it or lose it'. However, athletes are often very conscious that even a single training session dropped or day lost can result in detraining, but this is far from the truth. Detraining must be differentiated from *tapering*. Tapering involves the gradual reduction in training volume prior to a competition to give a physical and psychological break from the rigours of continuous training. Tapering allows muscle to repair microdamage caused through intense training (eccentric, or lengthening, actions especially, *see* Chapter 3) and to replenish the energy stores (muscle phosphocreatine and glycogen and liver glycogen). Interestingly, the gains made by top class training remain for some time. Research has shown, for example, that swimmers who reduce their training by 60 per cent for up to 21 days show no loss of fitness ($VO_2$ max), and actually improve muscle resistance to fatigue (due to lower blood lactate and increased arm power) (Costill et al 1985). Similar findings occur in running with a seven-day taper period in distance runners showing a significant reduction in 5k times (Houmard et al 1994).

Detraining sees the loss of the effects of training, but in a much slower way than injury or immobilisation. The detrained athlete shows muscle wasting (atrophy) and this becomes more noticeable in those who are highly trained because they obviously have more to lose. Atrophy is accompanied by reductions in muscle strength and endurance. Endurance begins to reduce after two weeks (Wilmore et al 2008) due to a reduction in oxygen usage capacity (a fall in both oxidative enzyme activity and muscle glycogen storage). Loss of cardiorespiratory endurance is greater over a similar time period than strength which requires only minimal stimulation to be maintained. Flexibility losses occur quite quickly. In a study looking at detraining in younger (<30) and older (>65) men, 8–13 per cent of strength gains were lost after 30 weeks to detraining (Lemmer et al 2000). However, power shows a more rapid reduction with similar reductions occurring in just four weeks of detraining (Costill et al 1985).

## INDIVIDUALITY

Training responses are not equal between individuals. We all have had the frustrating experience of someone starting at the gym a long time after us and improving more quickly.

Changes that relate to a specific person represent *individuality*. Each person reacts slightly differently to training stimuli due to differences in growth rate (which is genetically determined), and, for example, regulation of the cardiovascular and respiratory systems. Some people naturally adapt quickly (known as 'high responders') while others do not (low responders). In studies using the same training programme fitness levels ($VO_2$ max) can vary from 0–50 per cent (Wilmore et al 2008). The HERITAGE study in the late 1990s looked at family members' response to training (Bouchard et al 1999). Over 700 subjects completed a 20-week training programme and maximal oxygen uptake ($VO_2$ max) was measured together with risk factors for cardiovascular disease. Differences were showed to be related to genetics rather than age, sex or race.

## ENERGY SYSTEMS

In order to exercise you need energy, and this comes from food that the digestive system breaks down. The nutrients released are taken in the bloodstream to the working muscles, where enzyme action causes energy release. Some foodstuffs provide more energy than others. For example, sugars and fats are high energy providers, while fibre is a very low energy source.

When broken down, chemicals called 'phosphates' store the energy from food. These high energy phosphate fuels can almost be thought of as the 'petrol' in the body's 'engine'.

## ENERGY SOURCES

Phosphates are our energy 'currency' and we can 'spend' them in three ways when exercising. This gives us a choice of immediate, short-term or long-term energy supplies. One of the most important phosphate substances is *adenosine triphosphose* or ATP. This acts as a link between processes supplying energy and those (such as muscle contraction) which demand it. ATP is composed of a nitrogen substance called 'adenine', which is linked via high energy bonds to a sugar called 'ribose' and three phosphate molecules. When one phosphate molecule is removed from ATP, adenosine diphosphate (ADP) is produced and energy is released.

> ### Keypoint
>
> ATP (adenosine triphosphose) is made up of *adenine* (a nitrogen substance), *ribose* (a sugar), and three phosphate molecules.

### Immediate energy sources

A muscle can only store enough phosphate for about three seconds of maximal work. The phosphate used to do this is phosphocreatine (PC), sometimes called 'creatine phosphate'. Although this energy source is used up quickly (in about 10 seconds), it enables your body to react quickly and work maximally straight away, rather than waiting for energy to build up. For example, PC is used in the first few seconds of a sprint and during a low number of maximal repetitions in weight training. It is the energy source for power and speed rather than prolonged strength or endurance activities. PC can be reformed to be used again after about three minutes.

### Short term energy sources (the lactic acid system)

If exercise continues, PC stores quickly deplete, forcing muscles to use sugars (glycogen) for energy. This new process is termed *glycolysis*, and enables the muscles to continue to perform intense work – at a price. The price is lactic acid (also called 'lactate'), formed as a waste product, which interferes with the working of the muscle. This causes the muscle to ache and continuing the exercise eventually becomes too painful. The build-up of lactic acid is one of the sources of the 'burn' that is familiar to many sportsmen. The build-up of lactic acid limits the usefulness of this short term energy supply to about two minutes.

Both glycolysis and the PC system supply energy without using oxygen and are therefore described as *anaerobic*. Normally, at rest the concentration of lactic acid in the body is 0.5–2.2 units (mmol) per kilogram of muscle tissue. After heavy exercise, this concentration may increase to as much as 20–25 units as fatigue sets in (Mainwood and Renaud 1985). As the intensity of short-term exercise increases, the amount of lactate in the blood increases proportionally.

A graph of blood lactate plotted against exercise intensity (the *lactate accumulation curve*) shows a smooth line, with two distinct changes in gradient or 'breaks'. The first break in the curve is called the 'lactate threshold' (LT) and is seen at exercise intensities of 50–60 per cent of maximum, and is the point at which lactate is detected in the blood. The LT is expressed as a fitness value (oxygen uptake or $VO_2$) at which 2.5mm of lactate appears. The second break, called the 'onset of blood lactate accumulation'

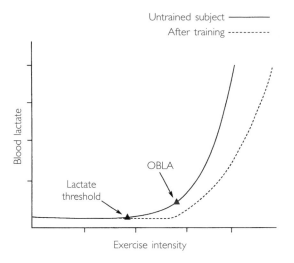

Untrained subject ———
After training - - - - - - -

Blood lactate

OBLA

Lactate
threshold

Exercise intensity

**Figure 3.2** The lactate accumulation curve

(OBLA) appears at intensities of 70–80 per cent maximum, and is similarly expressed as the $VO_2$ value when 4.0mm lactate appears. As you get fitter, it takes longer for lactate to build up and so the $VO_2$ value recorded at each point will be higher (*see* Figure 3.2).

Less lactate means less aching and the ability to exercise for longer, so your muscle endurance has therefore improved. This change is especially important in endurance events such as cycling and rowing, where muscle endurance as well as heart-lung endurance may be a deciding factor to optimal performance.

### Keypoint

Lactate threshold (LT) and onset of blood lactate (OBLA) are both measures of your muscle endurance fitness level.

## Long term energy sources (the oxygen system)

Long term energy supplies involve the use of oxygen from the air, and so are termed *aerobic*. Several fuels can be broken down in the presence of oxygen to form energy, including sugars, fats and even protein in some cases. This process is slower than both glycolysis and the PC system (*see* above), and it may be two to three minutes before the energy needs of the body cells are met through the aerobic system.

During this time the body, which is supplying its tissues with enough oxygen for resting requirements, must take measures to meet the increased needs during exercise. Heart and breathing rates increase, breathing becomes deeper and the blood flow to the working muscles improves. When all these changes have stabilised, you are said to have reached a *steady state*.

With training, these changes occur more rapidly because the systems involved become stronger. This is one of the health benefits of regular exercise. People in poor physical condition tend to take longer to reach steady state because their heart, lungs and muscles are not as efficient as those of trained athletes. A comparison between the three energy systems is shown in Figure 3.3.

In practice, the three systems work hand in hand. For example, when you start to exercise, the PC system and glycolysis supply the energy. The aerobic processes take slightly longer to come on line. In addition, the aerobic system does not stop immediately on cessation of exercise, but continues to work for a short while to recharge the other two energy sources. During this period lactic acid and other waste products are removed from the tissues so that they are ready for the next exercise period.

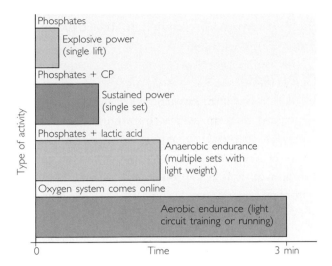

**Figure 3.3** A comparison between the three energy systems

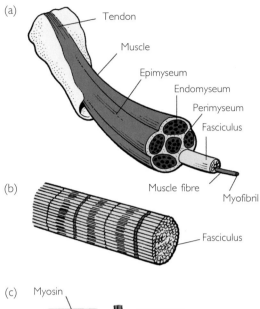

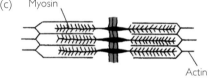

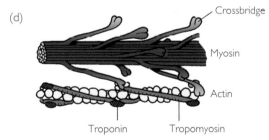

**Figure 3.4** Muscle under magnification

## MUSCLE ACTION

### MUSCLE STRUCTURE

If you take a small piece of muscle and magnify it many times (*see* Figure 3.4), you would see that it is made up of many long muscle fibres. This represents the muscle ultrastructure and each individual fibre is surrounded by a thin membrane (the endomysium), and in turn the fibres themselves are grouped together in bundles covered by another membrane (the perimysium). Finally, the whole muscle structure is encased in a sheath (the epimysium).

The fibres do not stretch from one end of the muscle to another, but are compartmentalised, with each fibre only about 10–12cm long. It is the muscle membranes that stretch the whole length of the muscle from tendon to tendon, intimately linking the contractile and non-contractile portions of the muscle. The whole structure is often referred to as the *musculotendinous unit*.

The muscle membranes are part of a larger network of connective tissue called *fascia* spreading across and between muscle groups, linking them together in fascial pathways. The combination of muscle fibre contraction and elastic recoil of the muscle membranes is important for the development of 'elastic strength', used in power activities especially.

31

Each individual muscle cell is surrounded by a further membrane, the *sarcolemma* (consisting of a basement membrane and plasmalemma), which is electrically conductive. The sarcolemma is not flat but folded, and the folds stretch out as the muscle fibre is stretched. *Sarcoplasm*, a gel containing the fuel stores (glycogen) and enzymes important to muscle contraction, is found inside the cell. Reaching inwards (laterally) from the sarcolemma are *transverse tubules*, each of which end on the muscle cell surface as a *lateral sac*. Also within the sarcoplasm is an intricate membrane, the *sarcoplasmic reticulum*, which consists of channels running parallel (or longitudinally) with the muscle fibres and winding around them.

Looking closely at each fibre we see alternating light and dark bands, corresponding to different muscle proteins. The light area is composed of a thin filament called 'actin', while the dark area consists of a thicker filament called 'myosin'. The two sets of filaments fit together like the fingers on two opposing hands, one set of actin-myosin fibres being called a *sarcomere*, and there are almost half a million sarcomeres in the longest muscles. The thick myosin filament has projections (cross-bridges) coming from it, much like the oars of a boat. The thin actin filament has a long *tropomyosin* filament wound around it and a globular *troponin* molecule is positioned over this area (*see* Figure 3.4). At rest the tropomyosin prevents (inhibits) actin and myosin from binding.

## CONTRACTION

Contraction of the muscle occurs when the muscle filaments move towards each other, and a whole sequence of events is required for this to take place. When you decide you want a muscle to contract, a nervous impulse (known as 'action potential') is sent from your brain down the spinal cord and along a nerve controlling movement (a *motor neuron*) to the muscle. One motor nerve may connect to a number of muscle fibres and this group is together called a 'motor unit'. At its end, the motor nerve enlarges to form an *axon terminal* which touches onto the muscle surface. Between the axon terminal and muscle membrane is a small gap called a 'synapse'. The electrical nerve impulse now causes the release of a chemical transmitter (acetylcholine or ACh) to flood across the synapse, in turn stimulating an electrical impulse to spread across the sarcolemma. As a result, stored calcium is released from the lateral sacs and passes down the transverse tubule to bind with the troponin molecule (*see* Figure 3.5).

This reaction causes the spiral tropomyosin to move deeper into the groove of the actin filament, removing the inhibition. Once the inhibition has been removed, contraction occurs spontaneously and the muscle filaments pull closer together, causing them to slide over each other and shorten the muscle.

The whole muscle contraction process uses energy, and rest is needed to recharge the structures involved. Calcium has to be moved out of the transverse tubule of the muscle and back into the lateral sacs. The filaments must then return to their original relaxed positions.

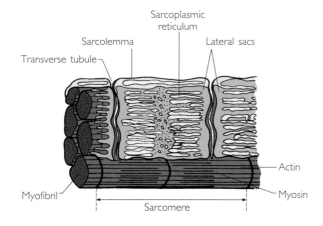

**Figure 3.5** Structure of a muscle – transverse tubule system

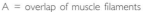
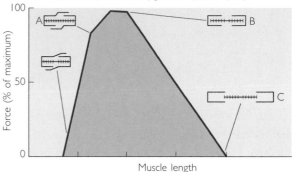

A = overlap of muscle filaments
B = maximum tension when filaments aligned
C = muscle overstretched (ligaments pulled apart)

**Figure 3.6** The length-tension relationship of muscles

## WHAT AFFECTS MUSCLE STRENGTH?

The amount of overlap that can occur between the sliding filaments of the muscle determines its contractile strength, and the relationship between muscle length and tension development is called the 'length-tension relationship' (*see* Figure 3.6).

When the muscle is shortened, the filaments are overlapped already and have little additional movement available to them. In the shortened position (inner range), therefore, the muscle is comparatively 'weak'. In the lengthened position (outer range), the filaments have pulled apart and the actin and myosin elements are disengaged. Again the muscle is relatively 'weak' – it can produce little active force through contraction – however, because the muscle is now stretched, it is able to produce some force through elastic recoil, known as 'elastic strength'. Therefore, the force in the outer range is mostly created passively through recoil, rather than actively through contraction (*see* Figure 3.7).

It is only in mid-range, when the muscle filaments are engaged but not overlapping, that maximal active force can be developed. Mid-range is the range that we use in our normal day-to-day activities, so functionally it is appropriate that this should be the strongest point in the available movement, and this is normally the resting length of the muscle.

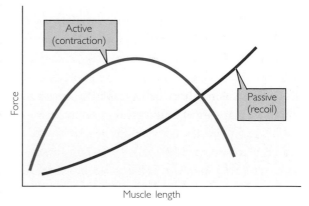

**Figure 3.7** Muscle recoil

## ELASTIC AND CONTRACTILE PROPERTIES OF MUSCLE

Muscle has three fundamental properties: contractibility, elasticity and extensibility.

### Contractibility

The contractile nature of muscle results from the movement of the sliding filaments within the muscle fibre, through which the muscle creates active force.

### Isometric

When the actin and myosin filaments come together, force is generated and the muscle shortens. If the muscle filaments shorten, but the external length of the muscle remains the same, the muscle tenses but the joint on which the muscle works does not move. This is an *isometric* or static muscle contraction. An example is holding an object in the hand with the elbow bent to 90 degrees. Isometric contraction stabilises joints and prevents movement, for example, isometric contraction of the transversus abdominis is used as a core stability exercise.

In many joints the muscles on both sides contract isometrically (called 'co-contraction') to brace the joint. Clinically it is the isometric endurance often referred to as postural holding which is important. Again, in core stability training a typical progression following low back pain, for example, would be isometric contraction of the muscle to familiarise the client with the action, and then repetitions, holding the contraction initially for 3–5 seconds building to 20–30 seconds over a period of some weeks.

### Concentric

When the muscle filaments shorten and pull the attachments of the muscle closer to each other, causing movement at the joint, the muscle contraction is then *concentric*. In our example above, instead of the arm being held still, the elbow joint bends (flexes). A concentric action tends to accelerate a limb, with the movement beginning slowly and getting faster. Very often, resistance training focuses on the amount of resistance that can be used, for example, the weight lifted or thickness of the band pulled. However, in many sports the action may be very fast so the rate at which the maximum force is applied (known as the 'rate of force development' or RFD) may be more important. If we take sprinting as an example, the athlete's foot may only contact the ground for about 100m and this is not enough time to develop maximum force. Training in this case would be better designed to improve RFD rather than amount of force. This type of sport involves explosive actions where power (rate of doing work) is more important than pure strength (ability to overcome resistance).

### Eccentric

Once the elbow has been flexed and the muscle filaments shortened, lowering the weight again involves the muscle filaments moving, but this time slowly paying out to control the joint as it extends. This is an *eccentric* action. This type of action is used to slow the body down and control movements, such as sitting down into a chair or walking down steps. Each time, the muscle filaments are sliding apart and the muscle is lengthening from a shortened position. Eccentric actions are actually stronger than concentric or isometric in that you are able to lower under control greater resistances than you can lift or hold. Force development depends on the speed of muscle contraction, and with concentric actions maximum force reduces as contraction speed increases. For this reason, in the gym people tend to lift heavier weights more slowly. Eccentric actions develop greater force with more rapid contractions. If you can't do a single chin-up in the gym, have someone lift you into a chin-up position and you will find that you are unable to hold yourself at the top of the movement or to lower yourself slowly (in both cases you may have to let go of the bar and drop to the floor), but you may be able to lower yourself the whole way down providing you do so quickly. The relationship between the amount of force that a muscle can create and the rate of contraction is called the 'force–velocity relationship' and is depicted in Figure 3.8.

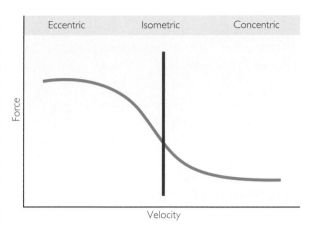

**Figure 3.8** The force-velocity relationship

> ## Keypoint
>
> In isometric contraction the joint does not move; concentric contraction causes acceleration and eccentric contraction causes deceleration.

## Elasticity and extensibility

*Elasticity* is the stretchiness of a material, or its ability to return to its original shape after a stress has deformed it. *Extensibility* is the give in a material, or its ability to lengthen when subjected to stress. An everyday example of elasticity is a rubber ball, and of extensibility putty.

We have seen that muscle fibres are compartmentalised by various sheaths. While the muscle sheaths cannot contract, they stretch, and they have important elastic properties. These elements of the muscle are known as the 'parallel elastic components' because they align parallel to the muscle fibres. The tendons at the end of the muscle are also non-contractile, but again they show elastic properties. These are the 'series elastic components', so-called because they are positioned before and after the fibres.

When tissue is subjected to stress, it gives or pays out and may not return to its original shape immediately. Rather than being elastic, the tissue is now said to be *plastic*, showing a more permanent change of shape. Human tissue displays both elastic and plastic qualities.

If a stretch is applied slowly and released slowly, muscle reflexes are avoided and any force produced by the muscle is purely passive through elastic recoil. This is important in posture especially. As we bend forwards to touch our toes, the back muscles (erector spinae) are lengthening eccentrically to lower the trunk. However, these same muscles are also being placed on stretch. When we begin to come back up from the forward bend position, initially there is no muscle contraction. We begin our upward movement purely through elastic recoil of the back muscles, a process known as the flexion-relaxation response. This mechanism is simply a way of conserving muscle energy, but it does illustrate the importance of maintaining healthy elasticity within a muscle. For example, if a person suffers from chronic low back pain, the flexion-relaxation response no longer occurs because the back muscles are continually in spasm and are unable to relax and stretch. The result is that the muscles have a poor blood flow because blood no longer pumps through the muscle as it contracts and relaxes and acids build up in the muscles, causing pain.

With rapid actions, muscle force is actually a combination of both elastic and contractile properties. When we lengthen a muscle its filaments move apart, ready to contract once more, and the elastic elements of the muscle are stretched. If this stretch is applied rapidly, a stretch reflex occurs in the muscle causing it to tighten and pull against the stretching force. If the muscle contracts immediately afterwards, the contractile force produced is a summation of contraction, elastic recoil and reflex mechanisms, and is far greater than if the muscle contracted from rest. We call this 'pre-stretching' and it is used to advantage in plyometric training where a series of jumps and bounding movements are used to build up 'elastic strength'.

> **Keypoint**
>
> Elastic strength comes from (a) muscle contraction, (b) elastic recoil and (c) muscle reflexes.

# MUSCLE FIBRES

## TYPES

All muscles contain fibres of different types. Slow twitch (type I) appear red under the microscope due to their high concentration of oxygen carrying *myoglobin* (an oxygen-binding protein) and are designed to contract over and over again without fatiguing. Fast twitch (type II) are white as they contain little myoglobin, and these give short bursts of power. Slow twitch fibres take roughly 110m to reach their maximum tension, while fast twitch fibres reach maximum tension in about 50m. Type II fibres can be subdivided into IIa, IIb (also called IIx) and IIc. Average muscle fibre make-up is about 50 per cent type I, 25 per cent IIa, 25 per cent IIx and 1–3 per cent type IIc (Wilmore et al 2008). Type I fibres are used for aerobic activities measured in hours, while type II fibres are used for anaerobic activity of 30 minutes (IIa), 5 minutes (IIb) or 1 minute (IIc). Type IIc fibres are thought to contribute to muscle adaptation. However, a person's muscles contain different proportions of fibres. Those who are good at endurance sports tend to have more slow twitch fibres in the leg muscles, while those who perform explosive sprints have more fast twitch fibres (*see* Figure 3.9).

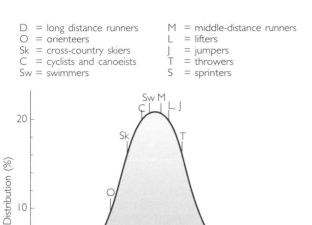

D = long distance runners    M = middle-distance runners
O = orienteers    L = lifters
Sk = cross-country skiers    J = jumpers
C = cyclists and canoeists    T = throwers
Sw = swimmers    S = sprinters

**Figure 3.9** Distribution of fast twitch fibre types

## RECRUITMENT

Motor units (neuron and muscle fibres it supplies) are not all recruited at the same time. Muscle fibres have nerves (motor neurons) supplying them, which vary in diameter with type IIb fibres having the largest and fastest neurons, IIa intermediate and type I small diameter and slower neurons. During resistance training, there is an order of fibre recruitment with the small diameter fibres being recruited first, followed by the intermediate ones. It is not until the muscle is subjected to high resistances (90 per cent maximum voluntary contraction, or MVC) that the fibres with the largest diameter neuron supply are actually recruited. This is known as the *size principle* of motor unit recruitment and it means that muscle contraction can be graded.

When a muscle gets stronger with training, two categories of change occur. Most people

assume that if you go to a gym and become stronger, it is because your muscles are becoming larger. These types of structural changes are called *'myogenic'* and they can actually take about six weeks to occur. Before that, strength increases are a result of *neurogenic* changes which are functional. Neurogenic changes include the body's ability to contract motor units together (*synchronously*) more effectively rather than in spurts with some contracting before or after others (*asynchronously*).

### Keypoint

Strength increases due to structural (myogenic) and functional (neurogenic) changes in the muscle. Neurogenic changes occur within the first 4–6 weeks of beginning a training programme with myogenic changes occurring after this.

## GROUP ACTION OF MUSCLES

A muscle can only pull, it cannot decide which action to perform. We produce an infinite variety of actions with a finite number of muscles by combining the various actions in different ways. This coordinated action of the various muscles working on a body part is called the group action of muscles (*see* Table 3.2).

When a muscle pulls to create a movement it is said to be acting as a *prime mover* or agonist. Most muscles can take on this function, depending on the action required and the site of the muscle. Other muscles may be able to help with the action but are less effective than the prime mover. The muscles that help are called 'secondary' or *'assistant movers'*. If we take elbow flexion as an

| Table 3.2 | The group action of muscles (example: elbow flexion) | | | |
|---|---|---|---|---|
| Prime mover (agonist) | Secondary (assistant) mover | Antagonist | Stabiliser (fixator) | Neutraliser |
| Creates primary movement (*biceps*) | Assists prime mover (*brachialis*) | If contracted, would oppose prime mover (*triceps*) | Stabilises or fixes bone origin of prime mover (*shoulder muscles*) | Removes unwanted action of prime mover (*pronators*) |

example, both biceps and brachialis can flex the elbow. In most circumstances the biceps is more effective and so acts as the prime mover, with the brachialis as the secondary mover.

The muscle that would oppose the prime mover if it is contracted is known as the '*antagonist*'. If we bend the arm, the biceps acts as the prime mover to create the power necessary to carry out the movement. To allow the movement to occur, however, the opposite muscle – in this case the triceps – must relax and in so doing acts as an antagonist.

Muscles do not simply create movements; they are also able to stabilise parts of the body or prevent unwanted actions by acting as *stabilisers* or fixators. In this case, the muscle contracts to steady or support the bone on to which the prime mover attaches. Take as an example the sit-up exercise. The abdominal muscles attach from the ribcage to the pelvis, so when they contract they move both body areas, tending to posteriorly tilt the pelvis and pull the ribcage down. To allow the abdominals to contract more effectively, we need to fix one body area to provide a firm base for the muscles to pull on. This occurs by the hip flexor muscles acting as fixators to stop the pelvis from tilting as the abdominals contract. In the

case of elbow flexion, mentioned above, because the biceps attach to the shoulder girdle, these bones must be stabilised to stop them sliding on the ribcage as the biceps contracts.

Many muscles can perform more than one movement. In the case of the biceps, for example, as well as flexing the elbow the muscle can also twist the forearm upwards (supination). If we want the biceps to perform just one action, bending the arm but not twisting it, other muscles must contract to stop the biceps from twisting the forearm. These muscles, which eliminate unwanted actions, are acting as *neutralisers*. As we saw above, the biceps muscle cannot decide which action to perform and which not to perform. Again it must be emphasised that a muscle can only pull: if we want to alter the action it produces, we must bring other muscles into play as neutralisers.

## Keypoint

*Prime movers* create an action, *assistant movers* help. *Stabilisers* hold a body part stable and *neutralisers* stop unwanted secondary actions which the prime mover can also perform.

## TWO-JOINT MUSCLES

Some muscles cross over two joints, and are said to be *biarticular*. The hamstrings, for example, attach from the seat bone (ischial tuberosity) to the top of the tibia. Because they cross both the hip and knee joints, they are capable of creating, or limiting, movement at both joints. Other biarticular muscles include the rectus femoris and gastrocnemius in the lower limbs, and the biceps and triceps in the upper limbs. Biarticular muscles have a number of important biomechanical features. First, because they pass over two joints, they cannot shorten enough to allow full movement at both joints simultaneously. For example, with the knee bent and the hamstrings relaxed at the knee, the hip can flex maximally, enabling the knee to be pulled right up onto the chest. However, with the knee straight and the lower portion of the hamstrings stretched, hip flexion is more limited. This limitation of movement at both joints is called '*passive insufficiency*' (*see* Figure 3.10).

If you stand up and flex your hip, you are able to bend your knee actively to touch your buttock with your heel. If you pull your hip into extension first, however, and try the same movement, you find that you are unable to touch your heel to your buttock. This is because in the first example the upper portion of the hamstrings was lengthened and the lower part shortened. In the second example, the upper and lower parts of the muscle are unable to shorten fully at the same time. This inability to create full movement at both joints simultaneously is called '*active insufficiency*'.

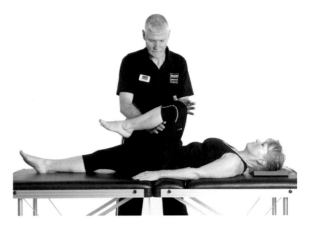

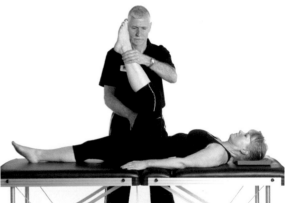

**Figure 3.10** Passive insufficiency

### Keypoint

A two-joint (biarticular) muscle, such as the hamstring or rectus femoris, does not permit full movement at both of the joints it spans at the same time.

| Table 3.3 | The two categories of muscle function: stabilising and movement muscles | |
|---|---|---|
| **Stabilising muscles (postural)** | **Movement muscles (locomotion)** | |
| **Characteristics** | **Characteristics** | |
| Deep | Superficial | |
| Predominantly slow-twitch | Predominantly fast-twitch | |
| Single joint | Two-joint | |
| Reduced activity (inhibited) | Preferential recruitment | |
| Lengthen | Tighten | |
| Light resistance | High resistance and ballistic | |
| **Correction** | **Correction** | |
| Improve tone and endurance | Stretch the tight muscles | |

| Table 3.4 | Examples of muscle types |
|---|---|
| **Stabilising muscles** | **Movement muscles** |
| Deep abdominals | Superficial abdominals |
| Gluteals | Hamstrings |
| Vastus medialis | Rectus femoris |
| Soleus | Gastrocnemius |
| Serratus anterior | Pectoralis major |
| Lower trapezius | Latissimus dorsi |

## MUSCLE IMBALANCE AND CORE STABILITY

Muscles can be broadly categorised into two types, depending on how they function in day-to-day activities (*see* Table 3.3). Some muscles, for example gluteals, act as postural or stabilising muscles, while others, for example hamstrings, act as locomotion or movement muscles.

## STABILISING MUSCLES

Stabilising muscles tend to be placed deeply within the body and act as postural muscles. Examples include the deep abdominals (transversus abdominis) and the deep spinal muscles (multifidus), as well as the gluteals in many situations (*see* Table 3.4).

These muscles are built for endurance and have many slow twitch fibres. They contract minimally, but hold the contraction for a long time. Unfortunately, in a person with an inactive lifestyle, or in someone who is active but has poor alignment, the stabilising muscles often have very poor tone and tend to sag. They almost seem to 'give way to gravity'. The tone is poor in these muscles not because they are weak, but because the nerve impulses – which control all muscles – find it difficult to get through to the muscle, and we say that the muscle has poor recruitment.

The poor recruitment of the muscle occurs because they have been infrequently used, and often because a person has had pain. For example, when a person has knee pain, one of the stabilising muscles of the knee (vastus medialis) will waste, and the same is true of other regions of the body. When we have back pain, our deep abdominals and our deep spinal muscles tend to waste and the nerve impulses to these muscles are reduced.

Because the muscles have not been used, we find it difficult to switch them back on – it is a case of 'use it or lose it'.

## MOVEMENT MUSCLES

Movement muscles, on the other hand, tend to be more superficial, for example the hamstrings on the back of the thigh and rectus femoris on the front. These muscles are very active in sport, being our sprinting and kicking muscles. They work over two joints, in this case the knee and hip, and tend to get very tight and powerful as they are recruited by hard and fast exercise and heavy poundages, such as in weight training.

Muscles of this type appear firm to the touch (palpation) and are often painful and hard after long periods of static posture, for example, in sitting or standing. They commonly develop focal pain areas known as trigger points (TrP). When touched firmly, the TrP can cause the muscle to contract rapidly and 'jump' or 'flick' painfully. In addition, pressing the TrP can cause pain to travel (refer) along the length of a limb. For example, a TrP in the buttock when pressed firmly can cause pain to spread across the buttock and down into the thigh. TrPs around the scapula commonly give pain across the shoulder and down into the arm. The pain can be intense and burning in nature. There are several methods of releasing a TrP, one of the most effective being stretching, either passively or using the PNF techniques. For further details see the *Complete Guide to Stretching* (Norris 2007) published by Bloomsbury.

### Correcting the imbalance

Because many forms of training tend to involve harder and faster movements, i.e. 'going for the burn', rather than slow controlled actions, for example yoga and tai chi, we end up with an imbalance of muscle length and tension around a joint. The imbalance leaves us with tight, strong superficial muscles on the one hand and sagging, poorly toned, deeper postural muscles. This gives rise to a number of postural problems and leaves us open to muscle injury through tearing. To correct the imbalance we must do three things:

1. Stretch the tight muscles
2. Improve the tone and endurance of the postural muscles by shortening them
3. Correct any alignment problems that have occurred (*see* Figure 3.11).

To begin with we often use core stability. This involves tightening the abdominal muscles using an isometric contraction to provide a stable base before we begin any stretching. If we fail to do this, as we stretch our alignment may be very poor. In Figure 3.10, the subject is trying to stretch the rectus femoris muscle on the front of the thigh by flexing the knee and extending the hip at the

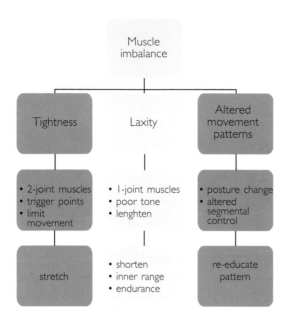

**Figure 3.11** Correcting alignment problems in the muscles

same time. To do this, the pelvis must remain stable and must not move. If the subject is unable to hold the abdominal muscles tight enough to stop the pelvis from tilting forwards, the stress from the exercise is thrown on to the lower back.

To correct sagging stabilising muscles in the muscle imbalance approach, we must shorten them, as excessive length rather than poor strength is their major problem. This is achieved by working the muscle only in its inner range (joint closed) rather than in its mid- or outer range (joint open). Inner-range work is paralleled with endurance exercise using exercises known as

'*inner range holding*' – literally taking the muscle into its inner range and building up holding time. Instead of adding weight progressively (2lb, 4lb, 6lb, etc.), as would be used in traditional weight training, we progress holding time (2 seconds, 10 seconds, 30 seconds, etc.).

Finally, when a person's body has been in a state of imbalance for a long period, their alignment and the way they move has been poor for so long that it has become a habit. These habitual movement patterns must be corrected because even when muscle strength and shortening has been addressed, incorrect movement patterns (known as 'movement dysfunction') can remain. Examples of such patterns include bending the back rather than the knees when lifting, hitching the hip when moving the leg sideways and shrugging the shoulder when lifting the arm into abduction. The underlying problem is one of coordination of one part (segment) of the body when moving another, and correction of this process is known as '*segmental control*'. We will look in closer detail at exercises to address muscle imbalance in the clinical chapters to follow.

## Keypoint

To correct muscle imbalance we must (a) stretch tight muscle, (b) shorten lengthened muscle and (c) improve body alignment and movement quality.

# METHODS OF EXERCISE PROGRESSION

4

We have seen that you need to overload tissue to enhance its performance. As the tissue improves, exercise must get harder to continue to sufficiently challenge the tissue. We call this structured increase in exercise difficulty 'progression'. When developing rehab programmes, your client may react poorly to an exercise, for example, if they have a joint swelling or muscle ache. This is an indication that the exercise is too strenuous at this stage of their recovery and it needs to be stopped and reintroduced later at an easier level, which is known as exercise 'regression'. Equally, when an exercise is too challenging the reaction is often simply to rest. Although the action should be stopped, total rest for a prolonged period is often detrimental to recovery. For this reason exercise regression must be mastered, your client being able to reintroduce an exercise at a lighter level to tax but not overtax the healing tissues.

## PROGRESSING AND REGRESSING EXERCISE

Most people think of progressing weight training (strength) by increasing the weight lifted, and progressing running (endurance) by running further or faster. In fact there are several ways to

| Table 4.1 | Factors to consider when progressing exercise |
|---|---|
| • Leverage | • Complexity |
| • Stability and base of support | • Gravity |
| • Energy systems | • Muscle work |
| • Momentum | • Range of motion |
| • Friction | • Starting position |
| • Speed of movement | • Resistance |

progress any exercise and the one we choose will depend very much on the injury, stage of healing and tissue condition. Table 4.1 shows some methods of exercise progression and although you will not use each factor with every exercise, let's spend some time briefly explaining how they work (Chapters 7–14 include examples of various exercises to illustrate each factor working).

## LEVERAGE

*Leverage* progresses an exercise by increasing the weight (load) of the object being lifted. When you move any part of your body the effective weight of the body part is greatest as the lift

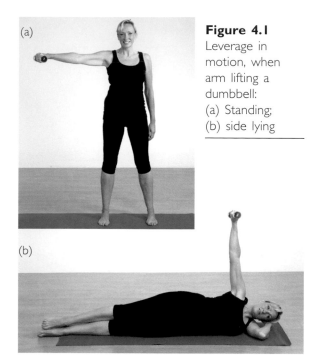

**Figure 4.1**
Leverage in motion, when arm lifting a dumbbell:
(a) Standing;
(b) side lying

(inner range) and fully open (outer range or end-range). If the point of maximum leverage corresponds to inner or outer range, it is often difficult for a client with weak muscles to move into this range. If they can move into the range, they may need to use a weight that is so light the rest of the range is not taxed. In modern weight training machines this situation is overcome by using *accommodating resistance*. In this type of machine a cable is used rather than a rigid bar and the pulley of the cable is not round, but shaped, to change the leverage. The shaped pulley is called a 'cam', and its effect on leverage is shown in Figure 4.2a, with an example of limited movement used in rehabilitation shown in Figure 4.2b. Accommodating resistance

gets closer to the horizontal and lessens as it gets further away from the horizontal. In Figure 4.1 the client is lifting a dumbbell out sideways. The leverage increases as their arm gets closer to the horizontal and so the exercise is harder at this point (a). By lying on their side (b) they perform the same movement (shoulder abduction), but now as the arm is lifted it is gradually moving away from the horizontal and towards the vertical. The movement is getting easier as the leverage reduces. To use leverage as a progression with this movement the sequence would be arm lifting in side lying, followed by arm lifting on an inclined bench and finally arm lifting in standing. At each point the same weight is lifted and the same action performed. The movement becomes progressively harder purely through changing leverage.

Remember that a muscle is strongest at its mid-range, when the joint is between fully closed

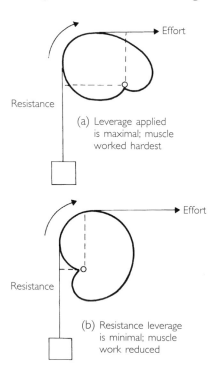

**Figure 4.2** Using the shaped pulley, or cam:
(a) Effects on leverage; (b) Limited movement in rehabilitation

alters throughout a movement, effectively making the weight lighter and heavier as it moves.

## STABILITY

Stability becomes more important in balance exercises. For example, standing on one leg (single leg standing) is important during the rehabilitation of both ankle and knee injuries. Stability is harder when the base of support is narrower. This means that a standing exercise performed with the legs apart is easier (more stable) than one performed with the legs together, and this in turn is easier than one performed standing on one leg (*see* Figure 4.3).

In addition the width of the base of support must be wider in the same direction as the movement which an athlete is carrying out. In Figure 4.4a the athlete is moving their arms from side to side (shoulder abduction) so the action is in a frontal plane. Stability is improved by widening the base of support in this plane by standing with the feet apart. In Figure 4.4b the action is forwards and back (shoulder flexion/ extension) and this action takes place in a sagittal plane. To become stable the base of support must be widened in this direction by placing one foot forwards and one back. In each case the area of the base of support is the same, but the direction in which it is widened changes.

Stability can also be challenged by making the base of support moveable (or labile). Using a balance board effectively moves the floor beneath your feet, challenging stability. The effect is to stimulate the body's balance sense and this relies on sensors both within the inner ear and the joints themselves. It is the sensors in the joint (proprioceptors) which can be impaired after injury due to swelling. When proprioception is poor the joint has a tendency to give way, and

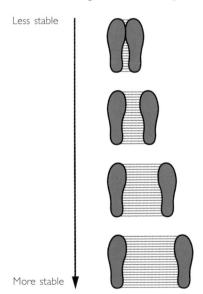

**Figure 4.3** Standing exercises with legs apart are easier to perform.

Less stable

More stable

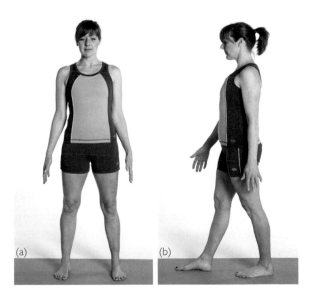

(a)  (b)

**Figure 4.4** Widening the base of support improves stability: (a) During shoulder abduction; (b) shoulder flexion/extension

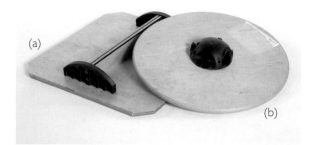

**Figure 4.5** Use of mobile surfaces for balance:
(a) Rocker boards move in a uniplanar motion;
(b) wobble boards move in a multiplanar motion

stability training has been shown to be the most effective way of improving it once more. Balance boards come in several types (*see* Figure 4.5).

Rocker boards have two half moon rockers beneath them and so move in only one direction (uniplanar). Wobble boards have a single half dome beneath and move in all directions (multiplanar) and as such are a progression in terms of stability. Where the dome is smaller the stability effect is greater (board is less stable). Foam rollers and cushions may also be used as moveable surfaces and are more yielding than boards. Vibration plates also challenge stability and may be used at varying speeds to have massaging effects on the body to stimulate circulation.

## ENERGY SYSTEMS

Energy systems refer to how the energy to perform an exercise is created by the body. As we have seen in Chapter 2 there are two ways: first with oxygen (*aerobic*), a method used for long runs and endurance events; second without oxygen (*anaerobic*), a method used for short, hard training such as sprints and weight lifting. Aerobic fitness is generally measured as the ability of the body to take up oxygen with maximal aerobic capacity ($VO_2$ max)

being the standard measure of cardiorespiratory endurance. Anaerobic fitness can be measured using a variety of tests, but the Wingate test (30 seconds maximum cycling) is probably the most commonly used test of anaerobic power.

It is important to use the same energy system in rehabilitation as is required eventually in sport. For example, in rehab a runner may begin by running a quarter of a mile and build up to half a mile and eventually 5 miles. We can see that the exercise is getting harder (progressing) and they are getting fitter. However, if they were a long jumper, a sport that requires short intense sprints, the training has not matched their sport (*see* training specificity below). We trained the athlete aerobically (5-mile run) when what they actually required was anaerobic training (reps of short sprints).

We can also subdivide anaerobic training between general anaerobic power (sprint) and muscle endurance (postural holding). In rehabilitation, muscle endurance is often more important, while anaerobic power is important for sports development. The ability of a muscle to hold a submaximal contraction is important for joint stability. Take the hip joint as an example. Following injury the muscles surrounding the hip (gluteus medius especially) may become lax. This muscle helps to hold the pelvis level on the weight-bearing side. If postural endurance in the gluteus medius is poor, when a person stands on one leg (injured side) the pelvis dips down. However, this may not be apparent for the first few seconds (or steps if walking). It is only when the muscle endurance is challenged by holding the action (single leg standing for 10–30 seconds) or repeating the movement (30 seconds of observed walk) that the impairment becomes apparent.

## MOMENTUM

Momentum is important when performing faster actions. Momentum builds up if you move your arm quickly, for example, meaning that it is difficult to stop moving suddenly. The heavier a limb is, the more momentum it will have, because momentum (described by the symbol 'p') is the product of mass ('m') and velocity ('v'), so p=mv. If you keep your arm straight and swing it from the shoulder, it has a certain momentum. Perform the same action holding a dumbbell and the momentum is dramatically increased because the mass (limb and dumbbell combined) has increased.

Momentum is important at the very start of rehab and at the very end. At the start a very stiff joint can often be freed up by using very gentle swinging actions of the limb. As an example, a stiff shoulder may be eased by using a pendular swinging action. Here, your client leans over a table and swings their stiff arm by using the sway of their body. The momentum of their arm keeps the action going without the need for muscle work.

At the end of rehab, the ability of muscle to work quickly enough to control momentum is important when performing cutting drills (changing direction rapidly) in sports such as football and rugby. An exercise can therefore be progressed by performing it faster or using a load and stopping the action, or changing direction rapidly to increase the effect of momentum.

## FRICTION

Friction may be used to both progress (make harder) or regress (make easier) an exercise. Often the resistance setting on home-user static cycles, for example, is friction based using either

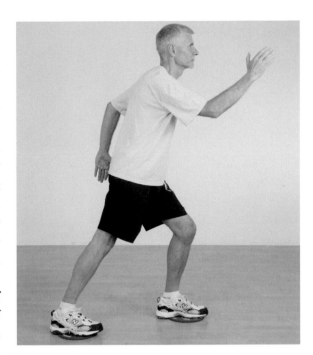

**Figure 4.6** Use a shiny surface to reduce friction while exercising

mechanical or electromagnetic braking, and *increasing* the friction setting makes the cycle harder to pedal.

Friction can also be used for sliding (*see* Figure 4.6). Slide training actions can be performed using a pair of thick socks on a shiny surface. In this case friction is *reduced* to allow free movement, for example side-to-side leg actions.

Increase friction for running by using a rope attached around the waist connected to a car tyre. The friction of the tyre pulled over a sports pitch significantly increases the difficulty of running (*see* Figure 4.7).

The advantage of using this type of resistance over a machine is that the tyre pull makes the action totally functional. The exact movement is rehearsed rather than one which is only similar.

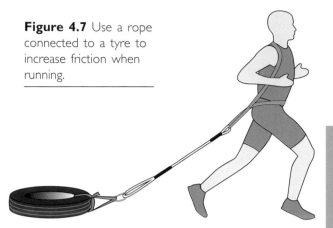

**Figure 4.7** Use a rope connected to a tyre to increase friction when running.

## COMPLEXITY

The complexity of an exercise is important to develop coordination. Use a simpler exercise initially as it is easier to understand, control and correct. Gradually, as confidence is gained use more complex actions.

Where a movement is complex it can be divided into several component movements. Each individual movement can be practised and mastered and then the components put together. This type of training is called '*part task*', and is a useful method for rehabilitation where individuals may not be skilled in movement production. However, it has a disadvantage in that sometimes putting the components together does not result in a smooth single action. Another method of learning a complex action is '*whole task*' training. Here your start with the whole complex action and accept that initially the performance of the action will be poor. Over time the action improves, as you remove those parts which are incorrect. The analogy here is of creating a statue; part task training would build it from blocks or bricks one at a time, while whole task training would begin with a solid block of stone and chip away, as with a sculpture, to reveal the whole statue.

Rehabilitation and sport make use of three types of part task training:
1. Segmentation
2. Fractionation
3. Simplification

*Segmentation* may be used where an action can be logically divided because the components have a definite start or finish. For example, a tennis serve could be divided into overhead throw of the ball, overhead swing of the racquet and step forward while bringing the racquet head down.

*Fractionation* is better used when the part tasks are carried out at the same time. For example, in a push-press-lift in the gym (pressing the bar overhead from the sternum) the knees must bend to absorb the shock of the bar as it descends. Both actions must occur at the same time but may be emphasised separately.

*Simplification* is making a complex task easier by taking one aspect of it away. For example, a squat action in the gym using a free weight bar may be simplified by performing the same action on a rack (perhaps a Smith frame), which allows the bar to move vertically but not forwards or back.

## GRAVITY

As we saw on pages 43–44, gravity forms part of leverage in exercise. Gravity can also prove useful in the early stages of rehab when it can be utilised to free off a stiff joint or to ease back pain. An excellent way to begin an exercise that would otherwise be painful is to allow the arm to hang freely while performing a shoulder exercise. When using pendular swinging, for example, a weight may be tied around the wrist to induce traction to the shoulder joint. The weight is tied rather than gripped to allow further muscle relaxation. Hanging from a high bar and allowing gravity to stretch the spine can relieve compression and pain on the lower back and apply traction to de-load the spinal tissues. Both types of exercise are examples of *gravity assisted* actions. *Gravity resisted* actions use leverage effects to make an action harder without the requirement for more weight to be lifted. For example, holding the arm out at a horizontal level requires a lighter weight to gain the same effect as actions that have your client holding the weight closer in. Gravity resistance of this type may also disguise the workload of an action. If we take a squat exercise as an example, the weight of the barbell placed across the shoulders creates a vertical force (compression) and a horizontal force (bending or torsion). Where the spine is held close to the vertical, the bending force is minimised and spinal alignment can be maintained. However, if the bar is allowed to move forwards, the horizontal component of its force increases, making its bending effect on the spine far greater. Where a large weight is used in a squat, horizontal movement of the bar by a few centimetres can increase the bending force on the spine to such a high degree that injury occurs.

Where the effect of gravity and leverage is not required, you may choose a *gravity eliminated* position. Now the action occurs in a horizontal (transverse) plane so the effect of gravity is constant across the range of motion. If we take the arm lifting (shoulder abduction) action described above, lying the client on their back allows the action to occur within a horizontal plane level with the floor. To do this some support is required to allow free movement and this can be supplied, for example, using a slide board or cloth on a polished surface (gym floor). Physiotherapy clinicians often use a method called 'sling suspension', where the arm is supported in canvas slings to allow horizontal movement without the client needing to hold the weight of their arm. This technique is useful where the arm is extremely weak (*see* Figure 4.8).

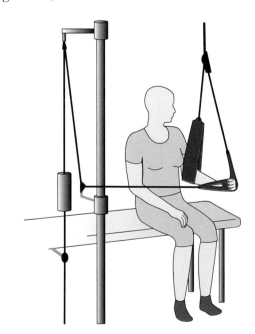

**Figure 4.8** The sling suspension method, useful for when a client's arm is extremely weak

## MUSCLE WORK

We saw in Chapter 3 that muscles work not just to lift an object, but also to hold it still and lower it under control. The lifting action is an example of a *concentric* muscle contraction, holding is *isometric* and lowering under control is *eccentric*.

The three types of muscle work can be further illustrated functionally when standing up and sitting down in a chair. As you stand up your thigh muscles are tightening and working concentrically, and your movement is accelerating. If you stop yourself just short of full standing and hold the position, the same muscles work isometrically. As you lower yourself down again back into the chair, the muscles are working eccentrically and you are decelerating.

We know that the order of strength reduces from eccentric to isometric and finally concentric (*see* Figure 3.8). You can illustrate this using a simple chin-up exercise on a bar in the gym. When you feel you can perform no more chins, step onto a bench and hold yourself with your elbows bent to 90 degrees. You will find that you can do this (isometric hold) although you cannot lift yourself anymore (concentric). Finally, when you can no longer hold yourself, you will find that you may be able to squeeze out a couple more reps if your training partner lifts you up and you lower yourself slowly (eccentric). This is a frequently used technique in bodybuilding and is known as a 'forced repetition', and the lowering (eccentric) portion of the movement is referred to as a 'negative rep'.

The three types of muscle work also have an important place within rehabilitation.

### Isometric actions in rehab

Isometric actions are used to hold a joint firm and prevent excessive motion. They are the *stabilising actions* that protect a joint. Building up the amount of time that a client can maintain an isometric contraction (holding time) is often important when re-educating stability following injury. For example, when treating low back pain a therapist often targets the deeper abdominal muscles, sometimes referred to as the corset muscles (transversus abdominis and internal oblique). The action used is a 'drawing in' movement of the abdominal wall (hollowing) rather than a sit-up movement. Initially clients may find this hard to achieve, but eventually they will perceive a mild contraction. To progress this rather than asking the client to contract their muscles harder, a therapist should build holding time, asking the client to perform the hollowing action for 3–5 seconds, then 10–20 seconds and finally 60–120 seconds.

### Eccentric actions in rehab

Eccentric actions are important because they often represent periods when the muscle is controlling movement of a joint as the body is lowering. It is during this type of movement that joints often give way, so training eccentric actions helps to prevent this while giving the client confidence. As an example, someone with knee pain often finds it far easier to go upstairs than to come down. Coming down is an eccentric action and each step takes longer than going up. We can train this action by progressing the lowering action using a step down from a shallow step (stand on a book), then a larger step (wooden yoga brick) and finally a single step on a staircase. The focus is to maintain lower limb alignment, keeping the patella over the centre of the foot throughout the movement.

Concentric actions are often the hardest to retrain when a muscle is very weak and, consequently, they are a source of considerable demotivation for clients. To retrain the actions, begin with eccentric actions and follow with assisted concentric. For example, following knee injury where a client finds it difficult to straighten their leg in a sitting position (sitting leg extension), straighten their leg for them and then ask them to lower it slowly, building up the time of lowering (3 seconds, 5 seconds, 10 seconds). Next, ask them to lift (knee extension) while you support the lower leg, taking some of its weight. Gradually ease off your lifting pressure as they are able to support more of their own limb weight.

## RANGE OF MOTION

Range of motion is how far a person is able to move a joint. Normally throughout the day we only use a limited amount of movement at our joints, because we rarely open (extend) or close (flex) the joint fully. This middle part of the joint's movement is called 'mid-range' (*see* Figure 4.9).

When you fully open a joint you are moving and stretching the muscles acting over the joint to *outer range*. When you fully close a joint and shorten the muscles, you are moving within *inner range*.

The key during rehab is both to use full range movements during training, and to match the movement range with that used in the activities your client will return to. For example, after an elbow injury you may be giving arm exercises to a javelin thrower. Because the elbow was injured there is a temptation to protect the joint and avoid full range movement. In the final stages of rehab, however, to prepare the athlete fully before competing, it is essential that they train the elbow to full outer range to mimic the stress on the elbow that will be encountered when they throw the javelin. Take as another example a patient recovering from hip surgery; they may be able to move their hip outwards (abduction) but might not be able to move to full inner range and hold this position (known as 'inner range holding'). This fact constitutes an important test for function because it shows that the client lacks sufficient muscle strength and control to stabilise the joint over time and, consequently, you must work to improve this.

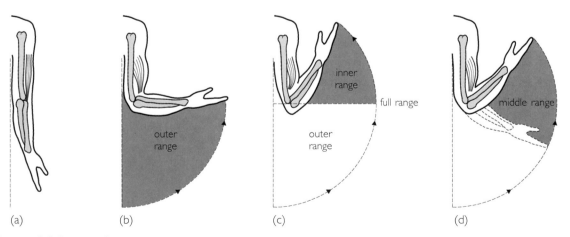

**Figure 4.9** Range of motion in a joint

## KINETIC CHAIN

Movements may be classified as open kinetic chain (open chain) or closed kinetic chain (closed chain). A kinetic chain is a chain of moving elements. In the case of the body it would be the bone components making up a limb. For example, the leg is a kinetic chain made up of the foot, shin and thigh bones.

### Open chain actions

An open chain action occurs when the end of the chain (known as the 'terminal joint') can move freely, i.e. when the foot is off the ground or the hand is off a wall. In a closed chain movement the end joint is unable to move freely because the foot is on the floor or the hand is on a wall and consequently that end joint is taking part of the bodyweight (*see* Figure 4.10).

Open chain actions are often rapid movements, such as punching and kicking, where the limb can move in a *ballistic* action. Here, muscles begin the movement and end it, but the middle part of the action also relies on the momentum of the moving limb; you are literally throwing the limb into the action. This requires large acceleration (speeding up) and deceleration (slowing down) forces at the beginning and end of the action and the muscle work involved is very subtly coordinated. If this coordination breaks down, injury can occur.

### Closed chain actions

Closed chain actions are generally slower movements requiring co-contraction of muscles, that is muscles on either side of the joint (agonist and antagonist) working together. In closed chain actions the joint is loaded (compressed) and the muscle work occurs to stabilise the joint especially.

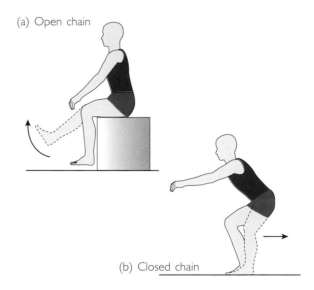

(a) Open chain

(b) Closed chain

**Figure 4.10** An open chain occurs when the terminal joint in the chain can move freely

### Definition

A ballistic action is a high velocity and high acceleration action giving a triphasic electromyographic (EMG) pattern. The EMG shows activity in the agonist, then antagonist, and finally agonist muscles once more.

During rehabilitation it is important to identify which actions will mimic the requirements of a body part during daily actions and sport and to select appropriate exercises to mimic these needs. In addition, because closed chain actions favour stability and open chain actions favour mobility, it is appropriate to select a starting position that favours the required result. For example, you may use a squatting action to stabilise the knee and a leg extension action to build muscle speed.

# SELECT APPROPRIATE EXERCISE COMPONENTS

We talk about strength exercise and stretching exercise as though each was completely separate. The fact is that very few exercises are completely pure and most have a variety of individual components. For example, the bench press exercise is categorised as a strength movement, but it also stretches the chest. For some individuals it may be better to reduce the weight (strength focus) and simply use a wooden pole to perform the action, making sure that the bar goes onto the chest completely (stretch focus). To categorise an exercise we must determine each component of the exercise, and for convenience we can describe them as 'S' factors (*see* Table 4.2).

| Table 4.2 | Exercise components: The 'S' factors |
|-----------|--------------------------------------|
| Stamina | Cardiopulmonary and local muscle endurance |
| Suppleness | Range of motion (ROM), static/dynamic flexibility |
| Strength | Concentric/isometric/eccentric |
| Spirit | Psychological aspects of fitness/injury |
| Speed | Rate/reaction time |
| Skill | Coordination/proprioception/agility |
| Specificity | Specific adaptation to imposed demand (SAID) |

## STAMINA

Stamina refers to both cardiopulmonary and local muscle endurance. Local muscle endurance is important in holding exercises and stability training. Cardiopulmonary fitness, the type used in aerobic training, is also important to restore following injury as further injury can occur when a person becomes fatigued towards the end of the game.

## SUPPLENESS

Suppleness or flexibility training is necessary to rehabilitation and vital to sporting performance. However, it is important to realise that there are several types of stretching, which target different anatomical structures. These include static (hold), dynamic (movement) and PNF (reflex) stretching, which largely target muscle. Joint mobilisation techniques aimed at the non-contractile joint structures (ligaments, fascia), and neural stretching aimed at nerves may also be included in the suppleness grouping. For further details on stretching see the *Complete Guide to Stretching* (Norris 2007), published by Bloomsbury.

## STRENGTH

Strength includes concentric, eccentric and isometric varieties (*see* pages 34–35). All are important components of an exercise and it is essential that the type of strength training is appropriate to the clients' requirements and the stage of tissue healing. We must also differentiate between requirements for strength, power and speed. For further details on strength training within sports *see Bodytoning* (2003, Norris), published by Bloomsbury.

## SPIRIT

Spirit is a term used here to describe the psychological factors that must be considered during rehabilitation. On the one hand these are important to general training for both health and sports performance. Factors such as motivation, how satisfied a person is with their own body and a positive outlook on life fall into this category. The way a person reacts to injury also has a psychological impact, depending on their psychological make-up, and factors such as personality type and anxiety/stress levels can all impact on recovery. If an injury is severe or puts an athlete out of a major competition, there may be a large emotional reaction and the psychological state may be similar to that of grief encountered in life threatening conditions (*see* Table 4.3).

In general, sports psychologists recognise three categories of response to injury in the athlete. Initially the athlete becomes *injury focused* and questions why and how the injury happened. This leads to *behaviour changes* and the athlete becomes agitated, feeling disbelief, and often dwelling in self-pity. Finally athletes move through these phases and *accept* the injury. They begin to be positive, engaging in coping mechanisms. Exercise is key during this latter phase as it gives the athlete the chance to participate in their own treatment.

## SPEED

Speed in this context also encompasses power. Speed is how fast we move (rate of movement) while power is how quickly we can move a resistance (rate of performing work), and both are important for explosive actions in sport and vital components of the final stages of rehabilitation.

| Table 4.3 | The psychological factors of injury |
|---|---|
| Denial | The unconscious refusal to accept facts: 'This cannot be happening to me, I've worked so hard in my training'; 'But I have a competition, I can't be injured now'. |
| Anger | Anger with themselves and others, making the athlete difficult to deal with: 'Who is to blame?'; 'They gave me the wrong exercise'; 'Those running shoes are to blame for this'. |
| Bargaining | Seek a compromise: 'Rather than rest, can I just run 3 miles instead of my normal 10?'; 'I'll go to the gym but I'll just use light weights – that will be OK won't it?' |
| Depression | Athlete withdraws and has long periods of silence: 'Just leave me alone'; 'What's the point?' |
| Acceptance | Athlete becomes emotionally detached from injury and becomes objective about recovery: 'I can't fight it, but I can work with it'. |

Another aspect of speed is *muscle reaction time*. This is how quickly you can contract a muscle, and is especially important to joint stability. If we take an ankle sprain as an example, the ligaments of the ankle have been overstretched and you need the muscles (especially the peronei on the outside of the joint) to compensate to keep your ankle stable on uneven surfaces. You can strengthen your ankle muscles using weight training, but this increased strength is of no use to you if your muscles do not contract quickly enough. For example, in the gym you may take 2 seconds to perform a heel raise action to strengthen your ankle. On rough ground, it may take only 0.25 seconds to sprain your ankle, so if you have only used weight training, your ankle muscles have not learnt to contract quickly enough. Once you have strengthened your ankle muscles you don't need any more strength, but you do need to maintain the strength that you have and make your muscles contract more quickly. This is the function of speed training.

## SKILL

Skill is important to all actions, but especially those involving complex movements. As we have seen, following injury you can develop movement dysfunction, that is you move differently to avoid the pain of an injury and this becomes a habit. Remember, in many cases it is more important to regain movement quality before movement quantity, and this is especially the case with the complex skilled actions seen in sport. Failure to address skill can place stress on previously healthy body parts and cause fresh injury. Going back to the example of the ankle injury shown above, a person will frequently walk with their ankle turning out after injury. If this change in walking is not corrected, it will place stress on the knee, hip and lower back, eventually leading to pain in these parts of the body.

## SPECIFICITY: MATCH THE SPORT REQUIREMENTS

When a muscle is strengthened, its make-up actually changes. We have seen that the muscle becomes larger and tighter, and there are alterations in the chemicals it contains. In addition, the way the brain controls the movement itself becomes smoother and more coordinated. All of these changes constitute what we call the 'training adaptation'. In other words, the changes that the body makes are a direct reaction to the training itself. The exact adaptation will closely reflect the type of exercise that has been used, and so we say that the muscle adaptation is 'specific' to the demands placed upon it. A simple pneumonic to remember is 'S.A.I.D.', which stands for *specific adaptation to imposed demand*. The change in your body as a result of exercise (*adaptation*) will always closely match (be *specific* to) the exercise you use (the *imposed demand*).

An example from general sport may make this clearer. Imagine two people who run marathons. They want to reduce their times and go for a 'personal best'. If one person trains by running long distances and the other by running short sprints, who will be more successful in reducing their times? The answer is the person who runs distances. This type of training more accurately reflects the actions required during marathon running. Marathon runners need endurance. Short sprints build mainly strength and speed, and so although the person using sprint training is getting fitter, the fitness is not the type required for the final marathon race. His body has changed (*adapted*) but these changes do not closely match those needed for running the marathon; they are not truly *specific*.

> ### Keypoint
>
> For an exercise to be truly *specific* it must closely match the action that we hope to improve.

As another example, let's look at the trunk. We need to know what function the trunk muscles perform, and then tailor our training programme to improve this function. Trunk muscle function falls broadly into two categories: support (stabilisation), which is important after injury, and movement, which is more important to sports performance. During stabilisation the trunk muscles work mainly isometrically to make the trunk more solid. During movement the muscles work concentrically and eccentrically to perform actions such as bending and twisting. If you perform multiple sets of sit-ups, you are actually working the movement function of the spine rather than the stability function. This has little effect on relieving pain as it is not specific to your immediate injury needs, and is more suited to later stage rehab.

Therefore, for an exercise to be specific to a sport it must match the movements involved in that sport. We can also match an exercise to the general day-to-day requirements of our client's body. In this case the exercise is termed *functional*.

For example, when you lift a heavy object such as a box you use your legs. We could argue that to strengthen your legs in the gym using a leg extension machine would improve your ability to lift the box. However, although training on this machine strengthens your legs, it does not rehearse the lifting action. Performing a deadlift action by lifting a barbell from the floor also strengthens your leg muscles. In addition, the deadlift rehearses the correct method of lifting a heavy object from the floor. Because it mimics the action your client will use when lifting a box each day, we say that the deadlift is a 'functional exercise', whereas the leg extension machine is a 'non-functional exercise'.

## Keypoint

A functional exercise mimics the day-to-day movements performed by a body part. It is 'real life' training.

# STRUCTURING REHABILITATION PROGRAMMES

# 5

We have seen how tissues heal (Chapter 1), the individual responses to injury of the most important tissues (Chapter 2) and methods of exercise and progression (Chapters 3 and 4). Now, we will look closely at how we can structure a rehabilitation programme to get your client back to full function quickly, safely and effectively.

## WORKING WITH HEALING

Healing involves the formation of a bridge across damaged tissue (*see* Chapter 1). As healing progresses, the tissue bridge becomes stronger and more able to handle the stresses and strains of exercise. It is now essential to stress the tissue enough for it to strengthen correctly. Too little stress on the tissue during the latter stages of healing when the tissue is remodelling results in it being weak. This is similar to exercising in the gym. To build strength, you need to stress your muscles using the resistance of weight or bands. If the resistance is too light, your strength will not improve. The same is true during rehabilitation.

We saw in Chapter 1 that healing moves forwards continuously, but for convenience can be divided into three phases. During these three phases the strength of the healing tissue changes.

Initially, during injury, tissues have torn or been bruised, so tissue strength rapidly reduces from normal. In this phase (acute) we must protect the damaged tissues from further injury and so exercise is not used – we say it is contraindicated. As the tissues begin to heal a blood clot forms and shrinks, so although the tissue is changing it is still weak and easily disrupted by movement. This represents the *lag phase* (*see* Figure 5.1).

Although time has passed since your client was injured and the tissues have begun to heal, tissue strength has not changed at all. Exercise on the

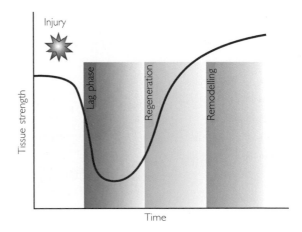

**Figure 5.1** The lag phase

injured area remains contraindicated until about 24–48 hours after injury. The time variation is dependent on the size of the injury.

> ### Keypoint
>
> Exercising an injured body part is contraindicated until 24–48 hours after injury due to the weakness of the healing tissues.

After this time we progress to the next stage of healing (subacute) where the blood clot is being replaced by fibrous tissue and the client is entering the phase of *regeneration* – as fresh tissue grows the area gradually becomes stronger. As tissue strength increases, the amount of exercise you are able to prescribe can increase. It is important that the pace of increase in exercise matches the increasing tissue strength. Too much and the new tissue can break down and re-injure, too little and the new tissue will be weak (*see* page 60 later in the chapter for details on how to monitor this process).

Tissue strength continues to increase until the point at which no new tissue is formed. From now on tissue strength slows, and the tissue begins to change to match that which existed prior to injury. This phase is *remodelling*, which occurs 4–6 weeks after the injury. Fibrous tissue never exactly matches the original tissue it has replaced, but most importantly full function will return with correct rehabilitation.

The local tissue changes largely dictate the pace of exercise progression. However, in addition to these local changes, whole body changes have also occurred. The quality and quantity of movement have both become impaired, and this is greater for larger injuries affecting a greater amount of tissue, and for long-term injuries which present a greater temporal (timing) effect. The body tries to protect the injured tissues by unloading them. This may mean an alteration in the way a body part is moved. An ankle or foot injury may result in your client laterally rotating their leg and rolling over the medial border of the foot, for example, to reduce the amount of ankle dorsiflexion required. A client with a knee injury may change the timing of their walk (gait cadence), putting their weight on a injured leg for less time than the uninjured one. Someone with a shoulder injury may change the way they lift their arm with the scapula moving more and the shoulder joint moving less, giving a change in scapulohumeral rhythm, with the shoulder appearing to shrug as the arm is lifted. These are all examples of changes in movement quality known as *movement dysfunction*.

> ### Keypoint
>
> Following injury, local tissue changes are paralleled by changes in quality and quantity of movement of the whole body.

Over time, the alteration in movement which occurs as a result of injury places greater physical stress (overload) on some tissues and far less on others. The result is imbalance of the tissues with some becoming weaker and underused and others becoming painful through overuse. In the example above, twisting the leg and roller over the inner aspect of the foot reduces stress on the injured ankle joint, but places greater stress on the inside of the knee. In time medial knee pain is often the result. Further up the chain of movement (kinetic chain) the rotation occurring in the low back can also result in asymmetry.

Additional changes occur as a result in alteration of motor control, such as poorer coordination and balance, and reduced speed of muscle contraction/reaction to externally applied forces. Psychological effects such as fear of movement and depression are also a consideration following long-term injury and exercise is an effective intervention in these processes as well.

> **Definition**
>
> Motor control is the organised transmission of nervous impulses from the motor cortex in the brain to the muscles resulting in coordinated actions.

The early stages of rehabilitation target the local tissue changes mainly, with whole body effects being the reserve of later stage rehab. However, putting some emphasis on the limitation of movement dysfunction in early rehab can prevent problems later. Use of crutches to support the limb and avoid limping is one example of the prevention of movement dysfunction by early intervention.

Early stage rehab (0–14 days) focuses on the basic fitness components of strength and flexibility (mobility). Later (14–28 days) speed and power training also become important and movements become more functional in that they mimic standard tasks seen in daily activities and/or sport. Final stage rehab (28 days onwards) can be almost entirely functional depending on the severity of injury.

## MONITOR DISCOMFORT AND PAIN

How do we match the rate of exercise increase with the changes occurring in the healing tissue? The key here is *feedback* from your client regarding their injury (*see also* Chapter 6). You must continually monitor the effect exercise is having on your client's injury – in short listen to their body and keep listening. At no time should your client be exercising through increasing pain. When your client begins rehabilitation they are exercising a part of the body that has been injured and not moved for some time. It is inevitable that they will feel some discomfort. When something is painful, OK it hurts, but how much? This is useful information to determine how to proceed with an exercise programme. Rather than have your client say 'a little' or 'a lot', we use a hospital-based pain scale (officially called a numerical rating scale). This is a score from 0 (no pain) to 10 (maximum pain) (*see* Figure 5.2).

Aim to monitor what your client feels at their injured body part throughout their rehabilitation programme. First, pain should not increase and, second, the intensity of the pain should not be great. Pain intensity (how painful the injury

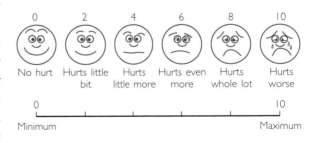

**Figure 5.2** The visual analogue pain scale (VAS)

feels) should be no higher than 5 or 6 on the pain scale. If it is higher than this, reduce the intensity of the exercise. If you have your client lifting weights, for example, use less weight or have them perform fewer reps. As your client exercises, if pain is caused by stiffness and new tissue stretching out, the pain should reduce with activity. Your client may score 6 for the first 2 or 3 reps and this might reduce to 4 or 5 as they get into the exercise. After a rest, when they perform their second set of an exercise the pain may once more reduce. This is a sign that the tissue is reacting in a positive way to the exercise and they can continue. However, if their pain score begins at 5 or 6 and increases to 7 or 8, you must stop immediately. Do not allow them to finish their set. Have them rest, and try again. If the pain stays at 5 or 6 and does not increase, you can continue, but cautiously. Increasing pain means that the exercise is putting too much stress on the healing tissues and they are likely to break down. Your aim should be to stress the tissues to get them to change positively (adapt) by becoming stronger or more flexible. If pain is increasing, the tissue is changing negatively (maladaption). It may be tearing, or becoming inflamed. Either way you are interfering with the healing process and risking a significant setback.

# TISSUE REACTION TO EXERCISE THERAPY

Following a rehab session, the next session must begin with a reassessment of your client's symptoms. Have they got better or worse? How did they react to exercise? The simple pneumonic SIN, which stands for severity, irritability and nature, can be helpful here. *Severity* of a condition can be determined by the amount of pain and typically this is done in hospitals on a pain scale (visual analogue scale or VAS), as described above. *Irritability* is how quickly a condition is stirred up, generally measured as the length of time your client does something before their pain increases (walking, bending, lifting, for example) and how quickly the pain settles once the activity is stopped. If your client has an injured knee which is painful after only two or three steps and takes 2 minutes to settle, it is more irritable than someone with a similar condition who can walk for 10 minutes before pain occurs and then settles within a couple of seconds. *Nature* of a condition reflects the stage of healing, whether acute, subacute or chronic. Also important is the type of injury – traumatic or overuse – and the amount of tissue damage – large (for example, extensive bruising to the hamstrings) or small (for example, a minor calf tear). Clinically we combine our impression of these three factors to limit treatment where SIN factors are high.

## Keypoint

Do not have your client exercise through increasing pain – stop immediately, have them rest and try again. If pain still increases, abandon the exercise.

## Keypoint

When assessing your injury's reaction to exercise, think 'SIN': severity (how bad is it?), irritability (how quickly is it stirred up?) and nature (what stage of healing is it at?).

## MEASURING EXERCISE INTENSITY

We have seen that training volume involves frequency, intensity and duration (*see* Chapter 3). Frequency (how often an exercise is practised) may be recorded in a training diary or treatment card, while duration is simply time. Intensity (how hard an exercise is) is more difficult to quantify. Two methods are commonly used to measure exercise intensity and whether you have it at the right level for your client: *rating of perceived exertion* (RPE) and *the talk test*.

## THE RATING OF PERCEIVED EXERTION (RPE) TEST

The RPE test is a rating scale which directly correlates to $VO_2$ measurement. That is, it accurately reflects changes, so the higher a score on the RPE test, the higher the $VO_2$ measurement and vice versa. The original scale described by Gunnar Borg in the 1970s scored from 6–20 (Borg 1970) and has since been modified several times, before its current popular incarnation, which uses a scoring system of 1–10. In statistical terms this is described as a category ratio scale and so the official title is the Borg CR10 scale, and it is often used to accurately measure exertion in the clinical environment in much the same way as the visual analogue scale (VAS) is used as a hospital measure of pain (*see* Figure 5.3).

The RPE test uses the client's own body sensations to monitor how hard they are working. Sensations of heart rate, depth of breathing, sweating and muscle ache all add up to our perception of how hard we work. Generally a score within the green zone of 3–4 (12–13 on the original scale) is seen as a light workload for rehabilitation.

| 0 | Nothing at all | |
|---|---|---|
| 1 | | How you feel sitting or simply standing |
| 2 | Weak | |
| 3 | Moderate | Exercise goal: How you feel when you exercise |
| 4 | | |
| 5 | Strong | |
| 6 | | |
| 7 | Very strong | How you feel when you really push yourself |
| 8 | | |
| 9 | | |
| 10 | Extremely strong | |
| • | All-out effort | You're unable to go on |

**Figure 5.3** The Borg CR10 scale: rating of perceived exhaustion

## THE TALK TEST

The talk test works on the fact that as exercise intensity increases we become more breathless until we are gasping and unable to speak. The change from easy conversation to laboured speak corresponds to around 50–60 per cent of your maximal heart rate (HRmax), and the test has shown to be an accurate measure of exercise intensity (Persinger et al 2004). Generally for early rehab a client's exercise intensity should always be low enough to allow them to comfortably hold a conversation.

## DEFINE OUTCOME MEASURES

An outcome measure is really a standard against which rehab can be measured. How do we know that the rehab program has been effective? We need to measure something before, perhaps during and certainly after the programme to track improvement. An outcome measure may be, for example, the number of painkillers that a client is taking – if this intake reduces it would indicate that pain is lessening. Other measures could include walking distance with a knee injury, or lifting capacity with a back injury. The key here is that the outcome measure has to be relevant to the client. It is no good saying that pain has reduced and so the client is discharged if the client's main concern is giving way in their knee, which has not changed. For this reason we normally use a Patient Reported Outcome Measure (PROM). These are normally standard hospital forms which measure changes in mobility, self-care, usual activities, pain and anxiety.

To really be specific to what is important to your client you may choose to let them define what they want measured and then allow them to measure it. The standard hospital test you would use to do this is the Measure Yourself Medical Outcome Profile (MYMOP, Patterson 1996). This questionnaire asks your client to define two symptoms which affect them (bother them) most, one activity that is important to them and then to rate their general feeling of wellbeing during the last week. The MYMOP form is available as a free download from this site http://sites.pcmd.ac.uk/mymop/files/MYMOP_questionnaire_initial_form.pdf.

You may feel that you do not need to be this specific if, for example, you are working with a personal training client. However, it is important to measure and record outcomes so you can review your work in the future. In addition, as part of good record keeping, the outcome you achieved should be recorded on your client's records together with full details of the rehab programme contents.

## OBSERVING MOVEMENT

When a movement is performed it is important to be able to observe what is actually happening to your client's body, because often the first appearance can be deceptive. Close observation and a structured assessment of movement is essential.

### JOINTS MOVED

Look at the whole movement and determine which joints are moving and therefore contributing to the action and which are not. If we take as an example someone standing up from a chair (*see* Figure 5.4), movement certainly occurs at the hips, knees and ankle as well as the shoulders. However, look more closely. Is your client moving their spine at all? Are they lifting their ankles from the ground so that movement occurs in the mid-foot? Is the arm movement just occurring at the shoulders, or are their elbows and wrists moving as well? Look even more closely at the shoulder. Is movement occurring just at the shoulder joint (glenohumeral joint) or do they shrug, in which case movement also occurs at the shoulder blade (scapulothoracic joint)?

### AXES AND PLANES

Once we know which joints are moving we need to find out how they move. For descriptive purposes the human body may be divided into three planes. The *sagittal plane* passes through the body from front to back, dividing it into right and left halves. The *frontal plane* divides the body into anterior and posterior sections, and lies at right angles to the sagittal plane. The *transverse plane* divides the body into upper and lower portions, and rests at right angles to the other two planes.

Each of the three body planes has an associated axis which passes perpendicularly through it (*see* Figure 5.5).

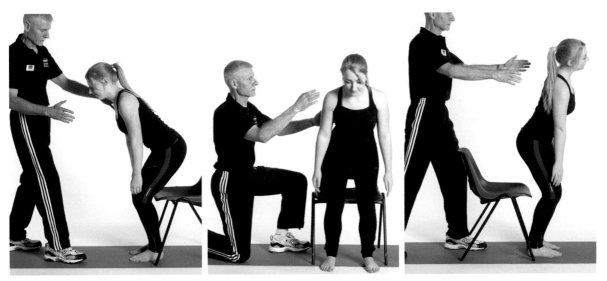

**Figure 5.4** Observing the movement of standing from a chair. View your client from the front, side and back to gain sufficient information about their movement pattern.

All body movements occur *in* a plane but *about* an axis. Pure abduction and adduction occur in the frontal plane about an anteroposterior (AP) axis; flexion and extension occur in a sagittal plane about a transverse axis; and rotations occur in a transverse plane about a vertical axis.

If the hip is bending, flexion is occurring in a sagittal (side) plane about an AP axis. Close observation indicates whether a movement is occurring about one (uniplanar), two (biplanar) or three (triplanar) planes. Functional movements are often not just restricted to one plane, but occur in several, and are said to be *multiplanar* occurring about an oblique axis.

This is important because most modern gym machines only work in uniplanar actions, which may not match your client's requirements. For example, let's say that we want to strengthen the knee and we decide that the movement required is knee extension. This occurs in a sagittal plane about a transverse axis. However, close observation may

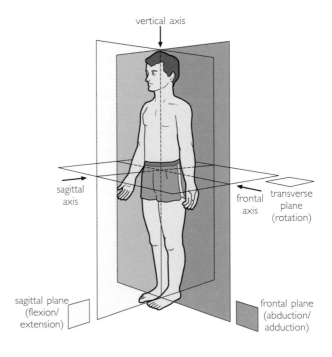

**Figure 5.5** The three planes of the body

show that your client's kneecap points outwards in sitting and forwards in standing, so some rotation is occurring, perhaps at the hip, knee or ankle. The gym machine will not recreate this, so we may need to chose a free weight activity instead.

## RANGE OF MOTION

We have seen that movement occurs through a motion range, with inner range being when the joint is almost closed (flexed), outer range when the joint is open (extended) and mid-range being the region between the two extremes (*see* Figure 4.9, page 51). Again we need to observe an action closely to determine which movement range is occurring so that we can recreate this during rehabilitation, or perhaps change/re-educate it. If we look at the knee joint in our chair squat example, the knee moves within mid- and outer range for extension. However, if we look more closely, does the knee stop moving when the leg is vertical or does movement continue with the knee joint hyperextending (known as 'genu recurvatum')? This action places considerable stress on the posteriorly placed knee structures, and if we were to use this action as an exercise, we would need to prevent hyperextension.

## MUSCLE WORK AND FUNCTION

We now know which movements are involved in the action, but what muscle work carries them out? Muscle work may be concentric to accelerate an action, isometric to stabilise, or eccentric to decelerate (*see* Chapter 3, page 34). In our chair squat example, the leg muscles work concentrically to lift the body from the chair. However, when we look closely, if the client has a poor fitness level, we may see a brief eccentric action if they rock backwards to pre-stretch the hip flexor muscles and gain momentum as they lunge the trunk forwards to initiate the action. The forward angle of the trunk is initiated by concentric hip flexor activity and maintained by eccentric action of the spinal extensors where the trunk bends (flexes), or the hip extensors where the pelvis anteriorly tilts. Typically both actions occur to some extent, but where trunk flexion is excessive pelvic tilt may have to be encouraged using a rocker board or sit-fit cushion.

We should also note asymmetry when viewing the action from the front or back as often clients may favour one leg or tilt the spine to one side, shortening the trunk side flexors on the concave side.

# EFFECTIVE EXERCISE TEACHING

6

## SKILLED MOVEMENT

Are rehab exercises skills? When you perform a leg extension action or balance on a wobble board, are you just using muscles or practising a skill? A dictionary definition of a skill is *proficiency that is acquired through training or experience*. Certainly your aim is to become more proficient at balancing on a wobble board through training, so the answer would be a resounding yes, rehab exercises are most definitely skills. However, we can dig deeper and see that there are different types of skills, and these differences are important to the way that we teach an exercise.

## SKILL TYPES

Skills may first be classified by how they are organised – as discrete, serial or continuous (*see* Table 6.1).

### MOVEMENT ORGANISATION

A *discrete* skill has a definite beginning and end. An example in rehab would be a sit-to-stand action. Once it is completed the skill has finished and you can go on to other things. If we put a number of individual discrete skills together as components of a larger skill, we have a *serial* skill. The order in which we put the components

| Table 6.1 | Classifying skills | |
|---|---|---|
| **Movement organisation** | | |
| *Discrete* | *Serial* | *Continuous* |
| Definite start and finish | Number of discrete actions linked | No definite start or finish |
| **Mental or physical involvement** | | |
| *Motor* | *Cognitive* | |
| Less decision making | More decision making | |
| **Influence of environment** | | |
| *Closed* | *Open* | |
| Predictable environment | Unpredictable environment | |

together is important because if we change it, the skill often degrades or fails completely. For example, a tennis serve consists of stepping back, reaching overhead, throwing the ball up, moving the racquet to the right point and striking the ball correctly. While each of these components can be practised separately, when we perform the full movement, if we throw the ball up before we raise the racquet, the tennis serve has failed. A *continuous* skill has no definite beginning or end but is repetitive in nature. Walking or running are examples of continuous skills. The end of the skill is dictated by the performer or the environment and the repetition is key to performance. A continuous skill may degrade due to fatigue, for example, because the technique is becoming poorer.

## MENTAL OR PHYSICAL INVOLVEMENT

The second way to classify skills is to describe how much importance is placed on physical movement or mental thought. *Motor* skills emphasise production of the movement itself, while *cognitive* skills focus on the decision-making process involved in carrying it out. An action such as a bench press in the gym is an example of a motor skill; the bar must be kept level and the muscle units synchronised, but there is little need to make other decisions. A cognitive skill focuses on strategy in sports or 'knowing what to do when'. All skills are in fact combinations of both motor and cognitive, but the proportion of each changes.

## INFLUENCE OF ENVIRONMENT

The final way to categorise a skill is to relate how the environment (external influence) affects it, and to measure the predictability of the environment during performance. An *open* skill is performed within an unpredictable (unstable) environment, for example, you could easily practise driving in a car on a treadmill in a lab. When you get out on the open road, however, varying roads, other traffic and hazards mean that your attention is pulled outside the car and your practise in the lab has not prepared you adequately. A *closed* skill occurs in a predictable (stable) environment, for example, we can return to the bench press action described above. You are relatively isolated from changes in the environment as you are lying on a bench and only moving part of your body.

We described the concept of training specificity in Chapter 4. With motor skills it is important that the skill type practised in training builds up to match the type of activity that your client will use in their day-to-day life or competitive sport. For example, if a tennis player suffers a shoulder injury, we should include strength training using weights as part of their rehab (discrete/closed motor skill). As we progress the rehab, speed and power activities to repetition should be included and could be practised in the gym using bands or pulleys (serial/closed motor skill). Eventually we can use ball throw and catch actions and throwing to a rebounder (open motor-cognitive skill) to introduce an unpredictable nature to the training, which more closely matches the skill type required in tennis and prepares the client for return to sport.

# HOW DOES A CLIENT LEARN SKILLED EXERCISE?

## THE INFORMATION PROCESSING MODEL

To understand how clients learn to perform a rehab exercise we need to spend a little time looking at how the body acts when presented with new information that demands an active response. We can think of the human organism a little like a modern machine, for example a computer. Information is presented as an *input* (your instructions to your client), they *process* this information (decide what to do and determine how to do it), and finally they produce an *output*, in this case an exercise. This is called the information processing model (*see* Figure 6.1).

It is important to note that a human does not simply respond to the information it takes in, but also processes it. As we will see later in this chapter, this implies that there in an interaction between currently held information (or knowledge) and new information (or the input).

The first stage is known as 'stimulus identification'. Imagine that you are at a party and everyone is talking. You are capable of hearing each voice but choose not to – instead they register as a general background sound. Then someone mentions your name and you look up – what has happened? Suddenly you have decided to tune into one sound rather than all the others. You have applied a technique called '*selective attention*'. This is your natural filter mechanism – it screens out things that you think are not important but tunes into things that you think are important.

It is quite possible for you to hear, see, feel, smell and taste several things at once. This is

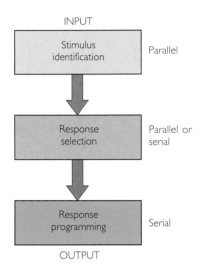

**Figure 6.1** The information processing model

> **Definition**
>
> Selective attention is a cognitive psychology term for a person's ability to pick out one stimulus (sound, vision, for example) within a field of numerous stimuli.

called '*parallel processing*'. Once you have received a stimulus that demands a response (for example, pain from stepping on a pin demands that you should move your foot to limit skin damage), you have then started the process of *response selection*. This stage can use both parallel processing or serial processing. We have seen that parallel processing means performing several things at once. Serial processing, on the other hand, involves performing actions one after another (in series). In the response selection phase of information processing, actions which are well practised may be processed in parallel, while unfamiliar or complex actions require more thought and need to be practised in series. Once we have determined what response to make (we are going to move our foot off the pin) we then need to *programme* the action in terms of coordination and muscle work. This process occurs in series.

At the response selection and response programming stages of the process there can be interaction with currently held knowledge. At the input stage, stimuli are detected and the interaction with current knowledge gives them meaning. So for example, when you are walking in the country and you see movement on the ground some distance ahead you may perceive this as a rabbit. When you get to the spot of ground you see that is was really an empty crisp bag that someone has dropped. The visual stimulus is the same in each case (the light reflecting from the bag into your eye), but the perception has changed. You perceived a rabbit because you compared the visual stimuli to memories of previous similar events and that was the one which seemed to match most closely.

At the response programming stage you are able to draw on stored movement programmes (or motor programmes). These are several individual movements that have been pieced together to produce a single sequence. So for example throwing a ball may consist of the individual movements: stepping (A), trunk twisting (B), shoulder movement (C), elbow movement (D), hand movement (E). The throwing action is a single programme which when begun runs A+B+C+D+E as a single sequence.

Importantly from a rehab perspective clients are often able to learn new actions if these are

### Definition

A *motor programme* is a series of nerve (neural) commands which when initiated results in a single sequence of coordinated movements.

linked to familiar movements. For example, if we are trying to teach abdominal hollowing as part of a core training programme, the action is quite difficult to understand for someone unfamiliar with exercise. Saying 'pull your tummy in as though you were trying to squeeze into a tight pair of jeans' links to a motor programme that the client is already familiar with rather than having to learn an entirely new muscle action.

Because several *simple* tasks can be processed in parallel while only one more *complex* task can be processed at a time, a bottleneck is created (*see* Figure 6.2).

This means that a complex action must be completed before another can begin. As many new exercise actions are complex for a client when they first begin to learn, it is important to limit

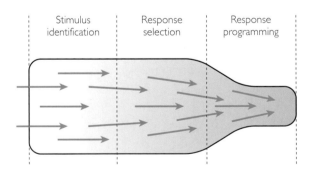

**Figure 6.2** Information processing 'bottleneck'

the number of movements learnt. Failure to do this results in actions interfering with each other and also degrading. The answer is to keep things simple in the early stages of teaching an exercise. Once the client becomes more adept at performing an action, it requires less of their attention and they may perform other actions in parallel. Let's look at the practical application of the information processing model in exercise therapy by reviewing techniques of motor learning.

## MOTOR LEARNING

Motor learning has been defined as a set of processes associated with practice or experience which leads to a relatively permanent change in the capability for skilled movement (Schmidt & Lee 2011). The learning process itself cannot be directly observed as it occurs internally, but we can judge the effectiveness of the learning that has occurred by observing results – in other words, how has the action improved as a result of the teaching and learning we have given? Motor learning is achieved through three interrelated stages (see Table 6.2).

| Table 6.2 | Components of motor learning |
|---|---|
| **Stage** | **Practical application** |
| Cognitive (understanding) | • Use proper demonstration and cueing<br>• Split complex actions into simpler subunits<br>• Short bouts of exercise with precision<br>• No home practice |
| Associative (effective movement) | • Link subunits together to form a single task<br>• Less cueing required<br>• Self-practice when client can identify own mistakes<br>• Increase repetitions |
| Autonomous (automatic action) | • Reduce attention to task<br>• Perform other actions while task is used<br>• Increase task speed |

**Definition**

Motor learning is the process of learning skilled movements.

## PERFORMANCE DURING THE COGNITIVE STAGE OF LEARNING

The first stage (cognitive) occurs when your client is finding out what is required of them and for this reason it is often referred to as the 'stage of understanding'. Here, your client is trying to form an idea of the whole movement. The process is very much 'thinking' (cognitive) rather than 'doing' (motor) in nature. Performance during the cognitive stage of motor learning is poorly coordinated, and your client will need to pay close attention to what they are doing. They must concentrate intensely and they can therefore tire easily. You can assist them by providing clear instructions and feedback to prevent them learning and repeating mistakes (your client may not be able to identify their own mistakes and so home exercise at this stage is inappropriate).

## Use proper demonstration and cueing

If we take a hip hitch movement as an example, although this action is familiar to you, it is most likely completely new to your client. If you demonstrate the action quickly, it will be difficult for them to work out what you are doing and therefore know what is required for successful performance of the exercise. If you are dressed in shorts so they can see the movement clearly, slow the action down and point directly to your hip and pelvis, telling them that your pelvis is lifting and you are keeping your leg straight, the action becomes easier for them to understand.

By making use of *cueing*, you are painting a mental picture of an action in terms which your client can easily understand. A cue (sensory cue) is really a way of communicating with your client other than by simply giving instructions. For example, an abdominal hollowing action may be cued by asking the athlete to pull the tummy button in (verbal cue) and showing them how to do it on yourself (visual cue). You could use the client's own fingers to feel their abdomen tightening (tactile or haptic cue). You can also use the intonation of your voice as you give instructions (auditory or verbal cue) to indicate the intensity of the movement and holding time, for example. Where you are demonstrating many exercises you can use several cues, a process called 'multisensory cueing'. For example, when lifting a heavy weight during bodybuilding, athletes often shout at each other (auditory), gesticulate (visual) and even strike each other (tactile) to encourage greater performance. Physiotherapists use a similar process of multisensory cueing in the rehabilitation of neurological conditions.

What you are really doing here is using environmental cues to help (facilitate) your client's

> ### Definition
>
> A cue is a signal that helps (facilitates) a particular action. Cues may be *verbal*, *visual*, *auditory* or *tactile* in nature. When a number of cues are used, the approach is *multisensory*.

learning. As they become more practised, these cues may no longer be necessary.

Often when teaching exercise to clients who rarely exercise it is important simply to get them to recognise or 'own' the part of their body that is injured. It may seem strange, but inactive individuals may not know they can pull their abdomen in, for example, and so have little chance of learning this action quickly. Given this, and the fact that they are in pain, you will need to give them as much information as possible to be able to regain control of their body so that they may participate in the rehabilitation progress. One of the ways we can do this is to make them identify more easily with a body part by focusing their attention on something that is familiar to them. For example, rather than saying 'tighten your abdominal muscles' or 'pull your abdomen in' (both of which assume that your client knows where these areas are), we can say 'pull your tummy button in'. In coaching terms, this is encouraging them to better develop internal focus (their body) rather than an external focus (the environment).

Your client is really working out how they can move their body to perform the action. We say that they are developing *strategies* to perform the end result (goal). Sometimes these strategies work and will be retained, and sometimes they won't and they will be let go.

## Split complex actions into simpler subunits

By splitting up complex actions into more simple components, you are providing your client with more manageable chunks of information, which can then be pieced together as they progress. For example, have them initially learn a single leg hop and twist as a single leg balance. Once your client is able to do this, go on to teach them straight line hopping then hopping and twisting on the spot and finally hopping and twisting over a distance. Clients unfamiliar with exercise require movements to be split up into even more chunks and will need to spend longer learning each part. Clients who regularly participate in sport learn skills more quickly and therefore won't require the task to be split up as much nor will they spend as much time on each component (revisit Chapter 4, page 48 to review the section on complexity as part of exercise progression for a description of part task and whole task training in this context).

## PERFORMANCE DURING THE ASSOCIATIVE STAGE OF LEARNING

The second stage of motor learning is the associative stage, which is really the stage of *effective movement*. Here, your client will try to perform the exercise with more precision by refining it. It is as though the original clumsy action is 'whittled down' to a smoother defined movement. Importantly, through practice, your client is now able to recognise their own mistakes, and so self-practice (unsupervised home exercise) is now allowed. Their dependence on *external* cues, such as visual and verbal encouragement from you, now gradually gives way to the reliance on feeling when the movement is right. This type of feeling comes from proprioception, the ability to feel the quality of movement of the body, and is *internal* to them. Movements become more consistent and your client is now able to work on the finer details of an action. Because the exercise is becoming more refined and efficient, it is less demanding both physically and mentally and so your client will be able to perform more reps. Greater repetition enhances their improvement still further.

You have now linked the individual movement sequences that you used in stage 1 to give a longer skill sequence. The actions must still be slow and precise, with progression made only when the movement sequence is correct, since practising an incorrect action causes the movement to degrade.

## PERFORMANCE DURING THE AUTONOMOUS STAGE OF LEARNING

The final stage of motor learning is the autonomous stage, where the action seems to 'run by itself'. This stage is often called 'automatic' (or 'grooved' in sporting circles). Movements at this stage demand less attention to perform and so your client will be able to perform other actions at the same time. By focusing on other actions, we are increasing the emphasis on automatisation of the skill. For example, during ankle rehabilitation we may begin with ankle re-strengthening and progress to a wobble board. Initially your client has to focus on keeping the edge of the board away from the floor while maintaining their own balance (cognitive stage). With repetition their ankle becomes stronger, their balance improves and they are able to perform the task (associative stage). Now, we can ask them to stand on the wobble board facing a wall and to throw and catch a basketball against the wall. Because they are focused on not dropping the ball, the balance and ankle stability becomes more automatic (autonomous stage).

## MOTIVATION

Motivation is the process that prompts or drives a person to act. It has been defined as the *direction and intensity of effort* (Weinberg and Gould 2007). The *direction* of effort is an indication of how a client seeks or is attracted to certain situations, while effort *intensity* is how hard an individual is prepared to work in a particular situation. Importantly to exercise therapy, motivation is the process which sustains a behaviour. Three approaches are generally used within sports science: participant (trait) centred, situation centred and interactional (*see* Figure 6.3).

> ### Definition
>
> A *trait* (psychological term) is a persistent thought, emotion or behaviour pattern.

It is the *interactional* approach which is most popular and has most relevance to exercise therapy. This recognises factors that are relevant both to the individual (intrinsic) and to the exercise environment (extrinsic). Intrinsic motivational factors give self-satisfaction and enjoyment, while extrinsic factors focus on an outcome or an external reward such as a certificate or medal. Identifying the type of motivator that a client responds to enables the therapist to structure the motivation process into goal setting.

### GOAL SETTING

Rehabilitation progresses over a period of time, and so improvement is often difficult for a client to see. Day-to-day changes may be slow, but by monitoring every few days or each week, improvement becomes more clearly apparent. To maintain motivation it is important for your client to have clearly described aims which act as stepping stones on the road to recovery. These aims or desires for a specific action are called *goals*.

Most people can identify plenty of goals for themselves; they want to be pain free, they want to be strong, to run again, to sleep better, for

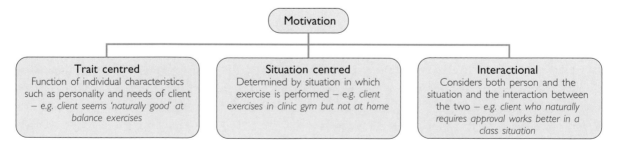

**Figure 6.3** Methods of motivation

| Table 6.3 | Goal setting in exercise therapy | | |
|---|---|---|---|
| **Outcome** | **Performance** | **Process** | |
| Focus on overall *result*, e.g. lifting an amount of weight by the end of a workout | Focus on *achievement* of a set standard, e.g. distance run | Focus on *quality* throughout an action, e.g. walking without limp | |

example. We can define goals as *objective*, focusing on attaining a specific outcome, for example, 'being able to lift 10kg for 5 reps', or *subjective*, general statements of intent such as 'wanting to do well'. In general goals may be categorised as outcome, performance or process (*see* Table 6.3).

*Outcome* goals focus on an overall result, for example, winning a race in sport or lifting a set weight in therapy. This is dependent on your own performance, but also on the (poor) performance of others, and this type of goal is less relevant to rehabilitation. *Performance* goals aim to achieve a standard independently of others, for example, being able to run a mile when recovering from a knee injury. *Process* goals focus on an action that must be maintained in order for a performance to be good, for example, walking with your foot aligned rather than turned out after sustaining an ankle injury.

### The SMART method

We need to set goals which stretch the client sufficiently but which are achievable. The simple pneumonic SMART helps with this process. An effective goal would be:

**S – specific:** It is no good saying to someone that they need to keep doing an exercise until their knee is better. The goal needs to be specific, perhaps lifting a certain weight or attaining a certain range of motion.

**M – measurable:** The goal must be able to be measured, otherwise your client won't know if they have achieved it. How do they know when their knee is better? Perhaps when they can climb ten steps, or hop four times, or twist on their fixed foot 30 degrees each way, twice, for example.

**A – achievable:** The aim of goal setting is to motivate your client. If the goal is set so far ahead (be able to run a marathon), it is not achievable in the foreseeable future and so does not motivate. The goal must stretch your client to be meaningful, but must not be so out of their reach that is cannot be attained.

**R – relevant:** The goal must be relevant to your client's requirements to act as an effective motivator. If they have no interest in attaining a goal, even though you think it is important, the goal won't be effective for them.

**T – timed:** Finally the goal has to be achieved by a certain date (be able to climb ten steps before the end of the month) so that it divides the rehab period into attainable chunks.

## FEEDBACK AND FEEDFORWARDS

### Feedback

Feedback is the process which tells a client how well a task was completed. In some tasks feedback occurs naturally or is *inherent*. In this case normal sensory information which occurs as part of the task gives the client knowledge of how well the task was completed. For example, if you ask your client to lift their arm up to the top of a cupboard,

EFFECTIVE EXERCISE TEACHING

you do not need to tell them how high to lift; if they touch the cupboard top, they have passed, and if they do not, they have failed. Feedback can be increased or augmented. Augmented feedback supports inherent feedback by giving more information. For example, if you place a bell or buzzer on top of the cupboard which sounds when they touch it, your client knows when they have touched the cupboard top (inherent feedback) but this knowledge is enhanced by the sound of the buzzer (augmented feedback).

## Feedforwards

Feedforwards on the other hand is predictive and provides information about what could happen in the future. As we have seen, feedback requires sensory information, which is processed by the brain and in turn the task may be modified to improve its accuracy. In contrast, during feedforward tasks there is an internal model constructed within your client's mind relating to accuracy of the task and no sensory information is required or processed.

The two methods exist at two ends of a continuum of control, with actions requiring feedback being slower but more accurate while those with feedforwards are faster but less accurate (Seidler et al 2004). Complex motor actions often require a combination of both feedback and feedforwards. Early in the learning phase more feedback is generally given to improve a client's accuracy. Once they are practised and have built their own internal model of accuracy, the task may be speeded up.

### Clinical scenario – using feedback in exercise therapy

When conducting back rehabilitation you can use feedback and feedforwards mechanisms. The deep abdominal muscles (transversus and multifidus) are used to enhance back stability. These muscles normally work automatically during actions that place stress onto the spine but can stop working following injury. To restore their function we begin retraining them by getting the client to contract them voluntarily and through the use of many different types of augmented *feedback* such as touch, vision and voice. As rehab is progressed the action becomes more automatic and less feedback is required. The client is required to contract the muscle automatically and maintain stability of their spine while conducting actions such as throwing and catching. They must predict how much muscle activity is required to stabilise the spine and gauge this activity throughout the task. The requirement for increased speed of muscle contraction to maintain stability means that these processes are now reliant on *feedforwards* mechanisms.

# HIP AND THIGH

## 7

## FUNCTIONAL ANATOMY REFRESHER

The lower limb consists of the pelvis, thighbone (femur) and two shin bones (tibia and fibula), some of which you are able to touch (palpate), as shown in table 7.1.

At the front of the outer pelvis is the *anterior superior iliac spine (ASIS)* which forms the attachment of the strap-like *sartorius muscle* passing diagonally across the front of the thigh to the inner knee. The ASIS is quite sharp and on very thin clients you may need to put a folded towel or pad beneath it when your client is lying on their front. At the side of the hip is the *greater trochanter*, an area which is covered by a balloon-like structure called a bursa. The bursa can swell if someone falls onto their hip, a common injury in skiing. Your sitting bone is the *ischial tuberosity* which forms the upper attachment of the hamstring muscles at the back of your thigh. At the side of the knee, just above the joint are two raised areas. On the outside of the knee this is the *lateral epicondyle* and on the inside the *medial epicondyle*, each forming the base of attachment for the outer knee ligaments (known as the 'collateral ligaments'). The shin bones are covered by muscle except for the bump

| Table 7.1 | Palpable structures in the lower limb |
|---|---|
| **Anatomical structure** | **Common name** |
| Iliac crest | Rim of pelvis |
| Femur | Thigh bone |
| Tibia | Inner shinbone |
| Fibula | Outer shinbone |
| Anterior or posterior superior iliac spine (ASIS/PSIS) | Sharp point at front of pelvis |
| Greater trochanter | Knobble on side of hip |
| Ischial tuberosity | Sitting bone |
| Lateral epicondyle | Raised area above outside of knee joint |
| Medial epicondyle | Raised area above inside of knee joint |
| Patella | Kneecap |
| Tibial tuberosity | Bump below the kneecap |
| Tibial crest | Sharp rim of shinbone |
| Lateral malleolus | Outer ankle bone |
| Medial malleolus | Inner ankle bone |
| Calcaneus | Heel bone |
| Tubercle of navicular | Highest point of inner foot arch |

beneath the kneecap, the *tibial tuberosity*, which forms the attachment of the patellar tendon, and the sharp front edge of the shin, the *tibial crest*.

The ankle bones (*lateral* and *medial malleolus*) form the attachments of the ankle ligaments, which are commonly sprained in sport. The heel actually consists of two bones, the *talus* forming the *mortise* within the ankle joint and the heel bone proper, the *calcaneus*. The highest point on the inner arch of the foot (*medial longitudinal arch*) is the *navicular bone* which forms the keystone to the arch. These palpable areas, which are easily touched during massage, are often referred to as bony landmarks and are shown in Figure 7.1.

The front of the thigh is made up of the quadriceps, a group of four muscles which straighten (extend) your knee. One of this group, rectus femoris, straightens your knee, but also bends (flexes) your hip. It is the kicking muscle and is commonly injured with mis-timed, violent kicking actions. The back of the thigh consists of the hamstring group attaching from your sitting bone to the top of your shin (tibia). These muscles bend your knee but also extend your hip, so they are involved in running actions. They are commonly pulled, and often need clinical massage.

The inner thigh muscles (adductors) travel from the inner rim of your pelvis to the inside top of your thighbone. The outer thigh muscles (abductors) come from your outer pelvis to the outside of your knee (femur, tibia and fibula). The abductor muscles (gluteals and tensor fascia lata) attach into the iliotibial band (ITB) which forms the shallow groove down the outside of your leg along the trouser seam. This structure is often very tight in those who participate in sport and requires clinical massage treatment.

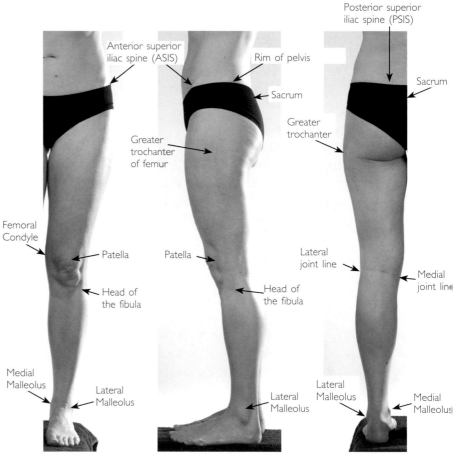

**Figure 7.1** The bony landmarks of the lower limb

## Exercise 7.1 Hip stability lying (clam shell)

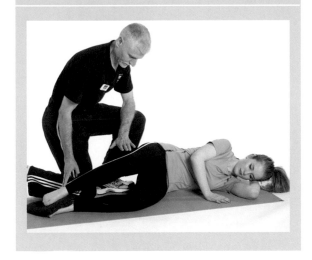

### Aims and usage

To work the gluteus medius muscle in isolation from the other hip abductor muscles, using closed chain non-weight bearing.

### Starting position and instructions

Begin with your client lying on their side with the right leg uppermost, their knees flexed to 90 degrees, hips to 45 degrees. Place a folded towel between their feet for support. The action is to lift the upper knee in an arc, keeping the pelvis still and the feet together. Encourage them to lift their knee as high as possible (inner range) and to hold the upper position initially for 5–10 seconds, building to 20–30 seconds (for muscle endurance).

### Variations

To emphasise the inner range position of the joint, begin with a cushion or block between your client's knees. Lift the knee from the block and lower back to the same position to work the inner range only, without work within the mid-range of movement.

### Points to note

As the gluteus medius function can be very poor, clients often try to rock their pelvis backwards to assist the motion. For pure isolation make sure they avoid this and focus on hip movement alone. Provide tactile cueing by tapping the muscle located just behind the greater trochanter of the femur.

## Exercise 7.2 Hip stability single leg standing with wall support

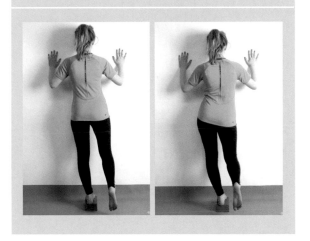

### Aims and usage

To focus on maintaining correct hip alignment in single leg standing

### Starting position and instructions

Begin with your client standing facing a wall and place both of their hands on the wall for support. Bend their right leg at the knee so that they stand on their left leg. Encourage them to focus on keeping both front hip bones (anterior superior iliac spines) horizontally level by asking them to draw or 'suck' in the hip at the side. This verbal cue is designed to avoid them pressing their side hip bone (greater trochanter) outwards.

## Variations

Move the right leg to the side (abduction) and back while maintaining the single leg balance position on the left leg. Placing your client's attention on the moving leg encourages a more automatic action of hip stability.

## Points to note

Encourage your client to take their weight over the outside of their foot to avoid a flat foot (pronated) position. Flattening the foot allows the knee to drift inwards, making contraction of the hip stabilising muscles more difficult.

**Exercise 7.3** Hip stability mini dip on block

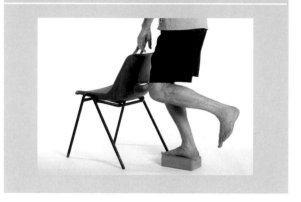

## Aims and usage

To maintain correct hip alignment in single leg standing while bending the knee

## Starting position and instructions

Begin with your client standing facing a high table, chair back or wall on which to place both

## Clinical scenario – hip replacement

Usually a physiotherapist shows a hip replacement patient exercises in hospital and then provides advice on how to continue with the rehab at home before discharging them. You may then see this person as a client perhaps one month after surgery. Their hip musculature will be very weak and they will need strength and stability work for the hip together with advice on walking correctly (gait pattern). Begin with isolation exercises such as clam shell (Exercise 7.1) and gluteal bridge (Exercise 7.14). Hip stability standing (Exercise 7.2) and hip stability walking (Exercise 7.5) begin the process of controlling the bodyweight over the single leg. Walking re-education can include inclined and declined walking (Exercise 7.13) and deep water walk (Exercise 7.12). Once hip stability has improved and your client can stand on one leg without their pelvis dipping (use the Trendelenburg test, see page 81) they can progress to more traditional strength exercises such as bench squats (Exercise 8.15) and lunge actions (Exercise 8.18).

Hip flexion (knee to chest) and hip adduction (crossing legs) should be limited, as this places stress on the joint which tends to separate the joint surfaces and can destabilise the replaced joint.

hands for for support. Instruct them to stand on a small (5cm) block placed beneath their right side. Encourage them to hitch their hip to bring both hip bones (anterior superior iliac spines) level horizontally by asking them to draw or 'suck' the hip in at the side. Maintain this alignment and then bend the knee on the right side to lightly touch the foot of the left side onto the ground.

## Variations
To offer less support, have your client stand side on to the table/wall and use one arm only for balance.

## Points to note
A firm book may be used as a block, but make sure they do not wear stockinged feet as they may slip on the shiny surface of the book: shoes or bare feet only.

---

### Exercise 7.4 Hip stability mini dip free-standing

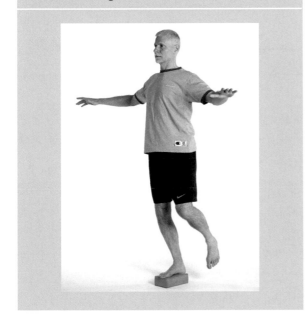

## Aims and usage
To focus on maintaining correct hip alignment in single leg mini dip

## Starting position and instructions
Begin with your client standing with the foot of their right leg placed on a block (5–10cm) or low step (10–30cm). Have them take their weight onto their foot and step onto the block, maintaining optimal hip and pelvic alignment. As they move upwards both hip bones should remain level horizontally and the hip on the right side should be 'sucked' in at the side. Maintain this alignment as they lower back onto the ground.

## Variations
Rather than lowering back to the same spot, ask your client to pause at the top of the movement and then lower their leg forwards so they step over the block.

## Points to note
The aim of this action is to reinforce optimal hip-pelvis alignment during movement. This feature of the action becomes harder (known as 'exercise progression') if the movement is slowed down, as stability has to be maintained for a greater length of time. If the total action (step up and step down) takes 20 seconds, there would be a progression on the movement taking 5 seconds.

## Exercise 7.5 Hip stability walking re-education

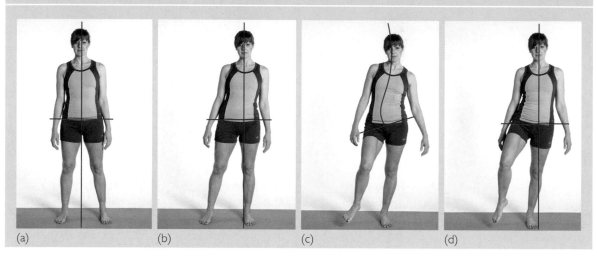

(a)            (b)            (c)            (d)

(a) normal standing; (b) weight shift to left leg; (c) pelvis dips down on non-weight bearing (right) side; (d) pelvis level in single leg standing

### Aims and usage

To maintain correct hip-pelvis alignment when walking

### Starting position and instructions

Begin with your client standing with their hands at their sides, or on their hips. Have them shift their bodyweight to the left and lift their right foot off the floor while maintaining a horizontal alignment of their pelvis. Place the right foot on the floor and take the bodyweight onto it, again maintaining correct alignment. Walk forwards slowly, step-by-step, transferring bodyweight from leg to leg while maintaining pelvic alignment.

### Variations

Perform the same exercise walking towards a mirror, but with the hands by the sides.

### Points to note

Using the hands on the hips provides tactile cueing of the pelvic position, while performing the exercise facing a mirror provides visual cueing.

## Exercise 7.6 Hip stability star tap

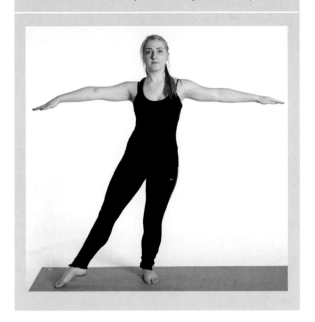

### Aims and usage
To maintain correct hip-pelvis alignment when walking

### Starting position and instructions
Begin with your client standing on their left leg with their arms outstretched to the sides. Have them take their bodyweight over their left side and lift the right foot off the ground, maintaining correct pelvic alignment. Tap the foot of the right leg forwards, then to the side, backwards, and then to the opposite side, crossing it behind the weight-bearing leg. Repeat the action for five cycles.

### Variations
Perform the same exercise while standing on a small (5cm) block and bending the weight-bearing knee slightly to touch the toes of the moving leg to the floor with each tap.

### Points to note
Make sure that your client looks forwards as they perform the exercise and not downwards at their hip or moving leg. Looking forwards forces them to depend on proprioception (joint feel) rather than vision for feedback.

## Exercise 7.7 Thomas stretch

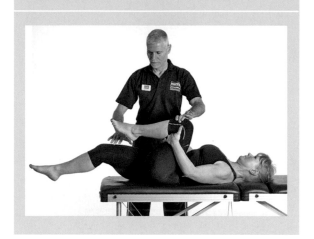

### Aims and usage

To place a passive (inactive) stretch on the hip flexor muscles

### Starting position and instructions

Begin with your client lying on a gym bench or treatment couch with their knees bent. Have them pull the knee of the left leg up onto their chest and hold it firmly in place. Gradually get them to straighten the right leg over the end of the couch and allow the leg to hang free.

### Variations

Allowing the leg to move outwards (abduction) takes stretch from the iliotibial band (ITB) and emphasises the hip flexors. Drawing the leg inwards (adduction) increases the ITB stretch.

### Points to note

For maximum stretch, the feet and shins have to clear the end of the couch. If they touch the couch, some of the overload on the stretch is reduced.

## Exercise 7.8 Hamstrings stretch using active knee extension

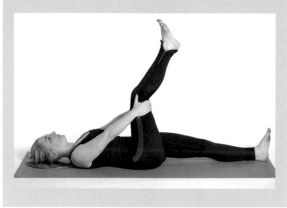

### Aims and usage

Lengthening (stretching) the hamstring muscles while contracting the quadriceps

### Starting position and instructions

Lie your client on the floor with their left leg straight and ask them to flex their right knee and hip to 90 degrees. Get them to grip their hands behind their right knee and actively straighten the leg using their quadriceps muscles. The knee should remain directly above the hip.

### Variations

Have them place their hand on the front of their leg and actively push it on to their hand using the power of their hip flexor muscles; at the same time, they should extend their knee. This causes the hamstring muscles to further relax through reflex action.

### Points to note

Rotating the hip (foot inwards or outwards) changes the emphasis of the stretch. Turning the foot inward (medial rotation of the hip) increases emphasis on the biceps femoris muscle, while turning the foot out (lateral rotation of the hip) increases the emphasis on semimembranosus and semitendinosus. Pulling the toes towards the body and/or flexing the neck throws stress on to the nerve (neural) tissues and away from the hamstrings muscles.

## Exercise 7.9 Knee extension using towel or belt

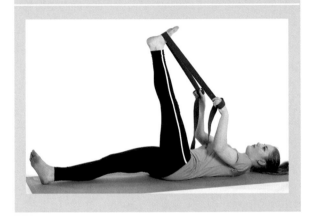

### Aims and usage

To use contraction of the quadriceps muscles to encourage relaxation of the hamstrings

### Starting position and instructions

Ask your client to lie on the floor with the right leg straight and flex the left knee and hip to 90 degrees. Hook a folded towel or yoga belt around their left foot, and have them hold one end of the towel in each hand. They then test their upper arms on the mat and attempt to straighten their leg by pushing their heel towards the ceiling. Ensure they keep the hip, knee and foot in a straight line.

### Variations

Instead of a towel, use an exercise band to offer resistance. Make sure that the band is in the centre of the foot rather than on the toes to guard against slipping. The action of pressing is now greater, as the band provides resistance, and so the activity of the quadriceps muscles increases.

### Points to note

By fastening the towel over their toes the client will pull the toes towards them. Combining this movement with flexion of the neck throws stress on to the neural (nerve) tissues and away from the hamstrings.

## Exercise 7.10 Hamstrings stretch – supported by door frame

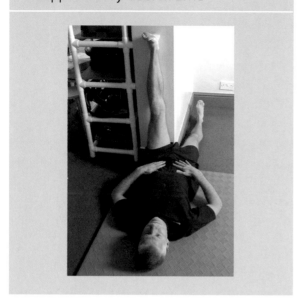

### Aims and usage
To perform a supported static stretch

### Starting position and instructions
Start by asking your client to lie on the floor in a doorway. Their hips should be level with the doorframe. Have them bend their left leg and place their left foot on the upright of the frame, keeping their right leg straight on the ground. They should then straighten their left leg, sliding their left heel up the doorframe as they do so.

### Variations
Have them move their whole body forwards or backwards so that the doorframe is at waist or knee level, which causes a greater or lesser amount of hip flexion and changes the intensity of the exercise.

### Points to note
Make sure that their heel stays on the doorframe to take the weight of their leg. If you find that their foot does not slide readily, ask them to keep their sock on to increase slip. Because the weight of their leg is supported they are able to perform a static (non-moving) stretch and hold the stretched position for longer periods. Have them begin holding for 20–30 seconds and build to 120 seconds. They should consciously control their breathing, focusing on exhalation (breathing out) to encourage muscle relaxation.

## Exercise 7.11 Rectus femoris stretch – standing

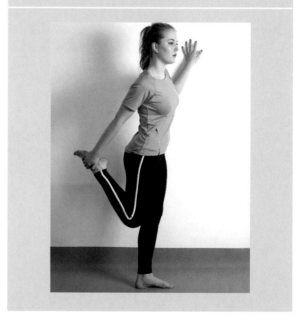

### Aims and usage
To stretch the quadriceps muscles, emphasising rectus femoris using movement at both the hip and knee joints

## Starting position and instructions

Have you client stand side-on to a wall with their left hand supporting their bodyweight. They should then flex their right leg and grip their ankle with their knee flexed. Next have them pull their right hip back into extension, while maintaining correct spinal alignment.

## Variations

Have them loop a towel around their ankle to reduce the amount of knee flexion and to allow them to pull in to further hip extension, which emphasises the upper portion of the muscle.

## Points to note

This exercise also stretches the femoral nerve travelling through the front of the thigh. If the client has suffered from back pain recently, a sensation of burning or tingling (pins and needles) over the front of the thigh may indicate that this nerve is tight or possibly trapped, which may require further treatment.

---

### Exercise 7.12 Deep water walk

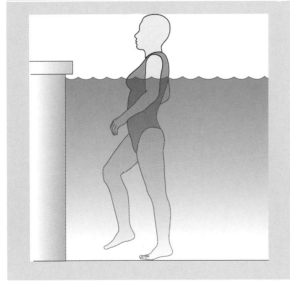

## Aims and usage

To provide joint unloading and muscle resistance to the lower limb

## Starting position and instructions

Begin with your client standing in chest-high water close to the poolside. Begin with them walking on the spot and progress to walking forwards, backwards and then side to side (sidestep). Initially the action is slow and controlled and may progress to power walking, the client taking longer strides and pushing against the water as they move.

## Variations

Have the client grasp a float in both hands, holding it vertically (its flat face *forwards*). As they walk forwards the float provides greater resistance to the water, making the action harder. Holding a float beneath each arm (elbow level) with its face *upwards* provides greater buoyancy, further unloading the lower limb joints.

## Points to note

Using deeper water further unloads the lower limb joints and provides greater resistance to motion as the body presses against a greater weight of water. Shallower water offers less resistance making movement easier, but also less limb unloading so more weight is taken through the joint.

## Exercise 7.13 Inclined/declined walk

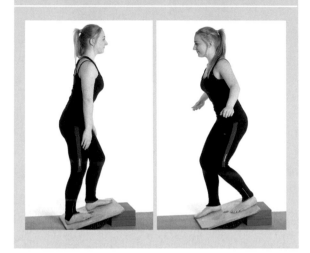

### Aims and usage

Use to prepare the lower limb for acceleration and deceleration loads

### Starting position and instructions

Begin with your client standing at the top (declined walk) or bottom (inclined walk) of a slope. Have them walk or jog down/up the slope, maintaining correct lower limb alignment. Ensure that the knee passes over the centre of the foot rather than the inside where the foot flattens, and that the pelvis is horizontal and does not dip. As they progress to the running action have them walk back up or down the slope to recover.

### Variations

To make this action easier (a process known as 'exercise regression') begin with a simple stepping action, having your client take one leg forward as they bend the knee of the weight-bearing side. They then return the leg and repeat the action using the opposite leg.

### Points to note

Clients often get pain in the knee when going down stairs or coming down slopes, when hill walking, for example, but not when going up. This is because the descending action depends on eccentric leg muscle work and occurs for a longer period than ascending, which is concentric work. Conversely, clients with back pain sometimes say walking up slopes is more painful than coming down. This occurs due to the forward lean (trunk and hip flexed) position of going up a hill. Declined or inclined actions initially using single steps and progression to walking and finally running can retrain these actions during rehab.

## Exercise 7.14 Gluteal bridge

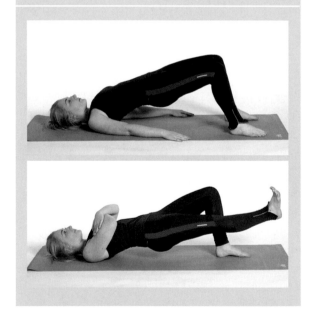

### Aims and usage

To strengthen the gluteal muscles using an isolation action

## Clinical scenario – hamstring tear

Hamstring tears can vary in intensity depending on the number of muscle fibres affected. Initial management is by the protect, rest, ice, compression and elevation (PRICE) method. Use cold packs to limit tissue damage within the acute phase of the injury and rest the leg in an elevated position (foot on a stool when sitting). Taping can help to support the injury by supplying compression to stop the spread of swelling in the early stages post injury and later to limit motion range as activities are begun. From 3–4 days post injury gentle muscle actions include bending and straightening the knee and light stretching using active knee extension. The knee extension using towel or belt (Exercise 7.9) provides a greater stretch and use the hamstrings stretch – supported by door frame (Exercise 7.10) to increase holding time of the stretch. In parallel with stretching, muscle strength and power must be increased using exercises such as deep water walk (Exercise 7.12) and gluteal bridge on ball (Exercise 7.15) using a varying knee angle. Build up speed using static cycling and controlled exercise such as a water kick (Exercise 7.24) prior to returning to progressive jogging and running drills. For details on the PRICE method, *see The Complete Guide to Sports Injuries* (Norris, 2011), published by Bloomsbury, pages 10–13.

### Starting position and instructions

Begin with your client lying on a gym mat with their knee bent to 90 degrees and feet flat. Have them place their arms to their sides, slightly away from their body. Ask them to tighten their gluteals (buttocks) and lift their body until their shoulders, hips and knees are in one line. They should hold the top position for 3–5 seconds and then lower.

### Variations

Folding the arms across the chest makes the exercise harder (progression). When the arms are at the sides they can use them to assist their legs in the lifting action by pressing into the mat. When they fold their arms this assistance is taken away meaning that the legs do all the work. To make the exercise even harder, ask them to straighten their right leg and lift just with the left. Initially have the heel of the straight (right) leg on the floor for balance and finally get them to lift the straight leg to the horizontal position so the bent (left) leg is taking all of the weight.

### Points to note

If lifting with one leg (single leg bridge), make balancing easier by asking them to place the heel of their bent leg closer to their centre line (the imaginary line drawn down the centre of the body).

## Exercise 7.15 Gluteal bridge on ball

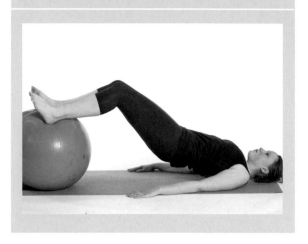

### Aims and usage
To provide gluteal muscle isolation on an unstable base

### Starting position and instructions
Begin with your client lying on a gym mat with their knees bent and arms by their sides on the mat. Place a gym ball in front of their feet. They should then come up into a bridge position and place first one and then both heels onto the ball. Have them press their heels onto the ball and lift their hips until their shoulders, hips and knees are in one line. Have them hold this position for 3–5 seconds and then lower back onto the mat.

### Variations
To increase the work of the gluteal muscles, have your client lift to a higher position (maximum) and then lower so that their hips are just off the floor. They should perform 10 reps before lowering their hips back onto the mat.

### Points to note
To make the balance easier to begin, have your client place their feet apart so they press into the top and sides of the ball. They may place the ball onto a plastic collar to stop it rolling until they gain good control of the action. Progress the action still further by having them perform a single leg gluteal bridge, keeping their right leg on the ball and straightening their left leg to the side of the ball so that they do not use it to lift their body.

## Exercise 7.16 Hip scissor side lying

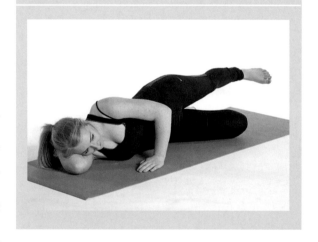

### Aims and usage
To work the hip abductor muscles with emphasis on the gluteus medius

### Starting position and instructions
Begin with your client lying on their right side with their right knee and hip flexed to increase their base of support and stop them rolling forwards. Have them bend their left arm and place their left hand on the mat in front of their

chest. They should then lift their left leg to 45 degrees, keeping it straight. Have them hold the upper position for 1–2 seconds before lowering.

## Variations

Turning the whole leg out slightly (lateral rotation of the hip) increases the emphasis on the postural portion of the gluteus medius muscle (posterior fibres).

## Points to note

If your client allows their leg to come forwards of their body line, the hip flexor muscles will begin to work, taking some of the emphasis away from the hip abductors. If you find the leg position difficult to control, practise the clam shell (Exercise 7.1) to begin. The clam shell action is easier because the bent leg is lifted (shorter level) and the foot is supported (reduced limb weight lifted).

---

### Exercise 7.17 Hip adduction side lying

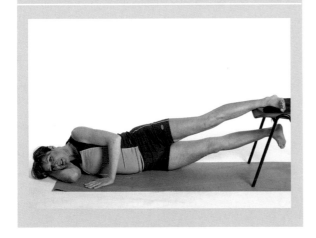

pause in this low position and then lift their right leg up again to touch the under-surface of the bench.

## Variations

Provide extra resistance for the right leg by having your client use a 1–2kg ankle weight.

## Points to note

The adductor muscles of both legs are working during this exercise. The right (lower) leg works during the scissor action (dynamic muscle work) while the adductor muscles of the left (upper) leg work to hold the body in position (static muscle work).

## Aims and usage

To provide intense work for the hip adductors muscles

## Starting position and instructions

Begin with your client in the side bridge position (right side down) with their feet supported on a gym bench or chair. Have them allow their right leg to drop down onto the floor, keeping it straight and moving from their hip. They should

## Exercise 7.18 Bent knee hip adductor stretch

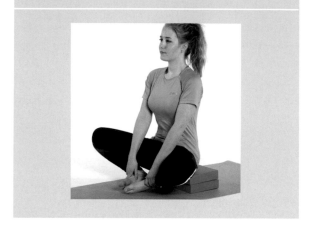

### Aims and usage
To lengthen the hip adductors muscles while maintaining spinal alignment

### Starting position and instructions
Begin with your client sitting upright with their spine aligned, knees bent and feet together. There should be a slight inward curve to their lower (lumbar) spine. If their spine is rounded at the bottom (lumbar flexion), have them sit on a folded towel or yoga block to improve their alignment. They should grasp their feet with both hands and gently press downwards using their elbows against their thighs. As they press down, ask them to focus on lengthening their spine and drawing their shoulder blades backwards (shoulder retraction). Have them hold the position for 10–20 seconds and then gently release. Perform 5 reps.

### Variations
If their back rounds excessively, have them sit with their back to a wall. This is a static stretch (stretched position held) but you may also use a PNF stretch, which tenses and releases the muscle. To do this have them pull their knees together (active hip adduction) against the resistance of their elbows. They should tighten the muscle for 5 seconds and then as they release, press their elbows downwards (passive hip abduction) and hold the lengthened position for 5–10 seconds.

### Points to note
Because the adductor muscles attach to the front of the pelvis (pubic bone), there is a tendency for the pelvis to tip *backwards*, rounding the lumbar spine. Sitting on a block tilts the pelvis *forwards* and prevents this.

## Exercise 7.19 Hip adductor stretch – wall support

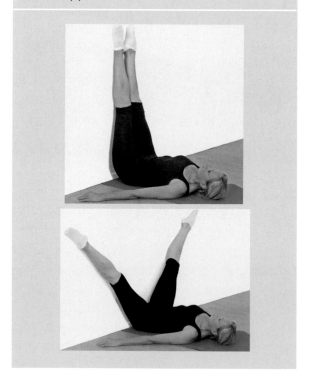

## Aims and usage

To stretch the hip adductor muscles including gracilis, which attaches below the knee

## Starting position and instructions

Begin with your client lying on the floor with their backside against a wall, knees bent up to their chest. Have them straighten their legs and rest them on the wall. They should gradually lower their legs out sideways (hip abduction) until they reach the point of maximum stretch and hold this position for 10–20 seconds.

## Variations

To increase the stretch have your client tighten their adductor muscles by raising their legs 5–10cm and then allow them to lower once more. This type of contract relax (CR) stretch aims to reduce the tone of the muscles, allowing them to relax further.

## Points to note

Although this is a stretching exercise, the legs are lowered by eccentric action (active paying out) of the hip adductor muscles. At the point of maximum stretch the muscles hold isometrically. To increase muscle relaxation, the weight of the legs can be supported on yoga blocks placed between the outer thigh and the floor.

### Exercise 7.20 Medicine ball flick

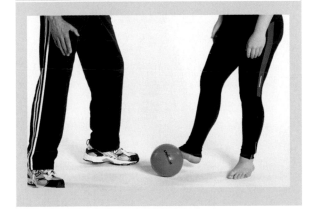

## Aims and usage

To apply multidirectional loading to the leg

## Starting position and instructions

Begin with your client standing side-on to you with a light (2–4kg) medicine ball at their feet. Have them place the *inside* of their foot on the ball and press it towards you (hip adduction). They should repeat this action, building up the speed to a slow and then more rapid flicking action over 10 reps. They should then rest and repeat flicking the ball with the *outside* of their foot (hip abduction).

## Variations

To build the ability of the leg to absorb sudden stress, have them gently tap the ball rather than flick. To flick, their foot is in contact with the ball as they start to move, to tap their foot is 5–10cm away from the ball when they move.

## Points to note

You may also have them perform flexion and extension actions by getting them to flick the ball with the top of their foot and aiming it forwards, or flicking with their heel and aiming it back. Pass the ball to them so they receive it from multiple directions to work for a greater variety of movements.

### Exercise 7.21 Standing pulley hip abduction and adduction

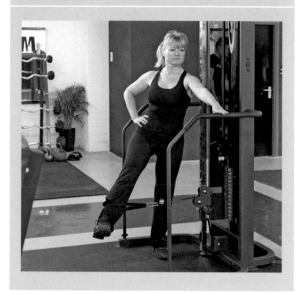

### Aims and usage
To strength the hip musculature in standing

### Starting position and instructions
Begin with your client standing side-on to a low pulley machine with the pulley strap around their ankle. They should take up the tension in the machine cable and keeping their leg straight, move it outwards in a scissor action. Have them pause in the upper position and then lower.

### Variations
To get your client to perform adduction, have them stand away from the machine with their feet apart (hip abduction), holding on to a support. They should then draw their leg inwards (hip adduction) against the resistance of the pulley.

### Points to note
Both legs work in this exercise. The moving leg works the hip muscles dynamically (muscles contracting to produce movement) while the standing leg works the muscle statically (muscles contracting to prevent unwanted movement). The standing leg muscles act to stabilise the weight-bearing hip.

### Exercise 7.22 Sitting pulley hip abduction and adduction

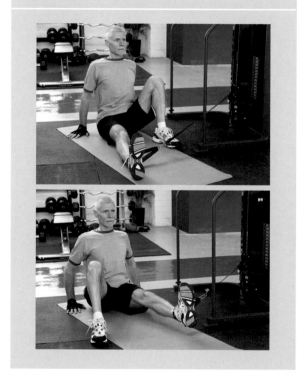

### Aims and usage
To strengthen the hip musculature in sitting

### Starting position and instructions
Begin with your client sitting side-on to a low pulley machine with the pulley strap around their

ankle. They should take up the tension in the machine cable and move their feet approximately one leg length apart. Keeping their legs straight, they then move their leg closest to the machine into adduction (legs together) to raise the weight, and then back into abduction (legs apart), controlling the descent of the machine weight.

## Variations

To work your client's hip abductor muscles, have them bend the knee closest to the machine and pass the machine cable beneath their leg to attach the strap to the ankle of their straight leg. They should abduct the straight leg (legs apart) and then move it back into adduction (legs together) under control.

## Points to note

Placing the strap over the ankle imposes a small but significant shearing stress to the knee. If this is painful for the client, have them place the strap above their knee. Doing this also reduces the leverage effect of the weight so you may need to increase the weight to work the muscle as hard.

### Exercise 7.23 Triplanar hip motion using pulley

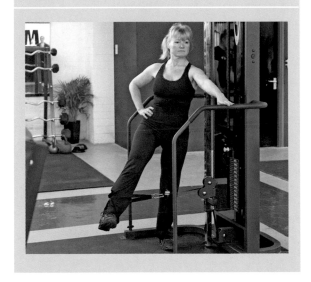

## Aims and usage

To work the hip musculature in multiple directions

## Starting position and instructions

Begin with your client standing side-on to a low pulley machine with the pulley strap around their ankle. Have them take up the tension in the machine cable and keeping the leg straight, move it outwards and forwards in a scissor action. Have them pause and then repeat the action movement, this time outwards and backwards.

## Variations

You may vary the speed of the action by reducing the weight and getting your client to perform a faster kicking action. Ensure that they control the descent of the machine weight: do not allow the weight to drop uncontrolled.

## Points to note

When a client performs speed training, their leg may move so rapidly that the weight is left behind and the machine cable becomes slack. For this reason as they speed up, monitor the cable tension and swap to resistance tubing rather than a cable machine if you detect any cable slack.

## Exercise 7.24 Water kick

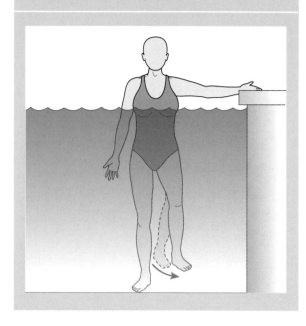

### Aims and usage
To initiate lower limb speed training

### Starting position and instructions
Begin with your client standing side-on to the swimming pool wall in waist-high water. Have them hold the poolside with one hand and move their leg forwards (flexion) and backwards (extension). Ask them to gradually increase the speed of the action until they are performing a kicking action against the resistance of the water. Have them move the whole of their leg, bending at both the knee and hip.

### Variations
• Vary the angle of movement by asking them to kick diagonally across their body (flexion-adduction) and out to the side (flexion-abduction).

• Limit the movement to one joint by asking them to hold their knee locked (hip isolation) or keep their knee in place and bend and straighten it (knee isolation).

### Points to note
The progression of this exercise is both motion range (how far their leg moves) and speed (how fast they move).

# 8

# KNEE

## ANATOMY REFRESHER

The knee is essentially two joints. The knee joint is formed between the thigh bone (femur) and shin bone (tibia) and officially called the *tibiofemoral* joint. The kneecap (patella) rests on the thigh bone (femur) and forms the *patellofemoral* joint at the front of the knee. Going back into our prehistoric past, the knee joint was actually in two parts. Now, the two have united into a single joint, but we still have an inner and outer knuckle, called condyles of the femur.

As with all major joints in the body the knee contains fluid and is strengthened by ligaments. However, the knee is unique in that it has an extra set of ligaments deep inside, called the *cruciates*. The ligaments on the inside (medial) and outside (lateral) of the joint support the knee in side-to-side movements, while the cruciates support it in forward and backward movements (*see* Figure 8.1).

The muscles controlling the knee have been described in Chapter 5, and are the quadriceps at the front, hamstrings at the back, adductors (inner) and abductors (outer) at the sides. The quadriceps are especially important following injury as they reduce their size (waste) very quickly. Within 48 hours of an injury that causes swelling in the knee, the quads can visibly waste. This occurs

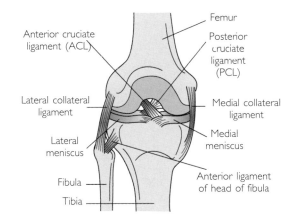

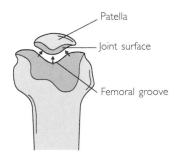

**Figure 8.1** The knee ligaments

much more quickly than simply through rest, and is the result of reflexes in the knee reducing the normal nervous impulses travelling to and fro from the joint. This type of muscle reaction is called *inhibition* and it affects a portion of the innermost quads muscle especially. This area is known as the vastus medialis obliquus (VMO) and is sometimes called the 'key to the knee' because it is important for controlling the position of the kneecap and locking the knee out straight. When the VMO wastes, the knee often fails to lock and can give way.

The knee joint condyles are rounded, but the surface they contact (the plateaux of the tibia) is flat. To enable a better fit, there are two extra pieces of cartilage, each called a meniscus (plural menisci), on the joint surface of the tibia. These are semi circles, and thinner on the inside than the outside. The inner (medial) meniscus is more often torn, and part or all of it removed surgically as a result in an operation called a 'meniscectomy'. Intensive rehabilitation is required following this type of surgery.

## Exercise 8.1 Knee brace

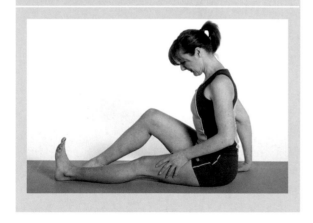

### Aims and usage
To encourage knee locking

### Starting position and instructions
Begin with your client sitting on a bench or the floor. Have them tighten their quadriceps muscles (the instruction 'lift your kneecap up' is a useful verbal cue) and press the back of their knee to the bench or floor. Have them hold the position for 10 seconds and then release.

### Variations
Where the knee has been swollen and won't straighten fully, place a folded towel between the back of their knee (popliteal region) and the bench. Have them press down to squeeze the back of their knee against the towel and compress it. Initially they should aim to hyperextend the knee slightly so their heel lifts from the bench by 1–2cm.

### Points to note
Following injury the quadriceps muscles may be *inhibited* or poorly *recruited*. Inhibition means that another nerve stimulus (usually pain or swelling) is cancelling out the stimulus the brain is giving to contract the muscle. Where this happens it is essential to reduce pain and swelling in parallel with trying to contract the muscle. Poor recruitment means that nervous impulses are finding it hard to get through to the muscle, normally after a prolonged period of rest in a plaster cast, for example. To contract the muscle it needs to be stimulated manually (percussion massage) or electrically (electrotherapy).

## Exercise 8.2 Straight leg raise

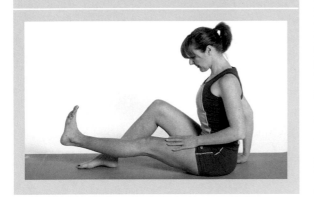

### Aims and usage
To maintain a locked position when the knee is unsupported

### Starting position and instructions
Begin with your client sitting on a bench or the floor. Have them tighten their quadriceps muscles and press their knee back to the floor to lock it out straight. They should then raise the whole leg by 10–20cm, holding the raised position for 5–10 seconds before lowering.

### Variations
Guide your client's leg by pressing into their heel and lifting your hand as their leg lifts. Take some of your client's leg weight as they lift (concentric action) and release as they lower (eccentric action).

### Points to note
Following injury the knee may lock when supported, but unlock slightly when lifted. This is called an extensor lag and can be quite subtle. To assess the knee, look from the side and compare the line of the thigh bone (femur) to the shin bone (tibia) when the leg is flat and when lifted.

## Exercise 8.3 Capsular stretch to knee

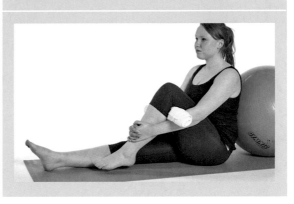

### Aims and usage
To stretch the knee joint capsule/ligaments and increase flexion range

### Starting position and instructions
Begin with your client sitting on the floor with their back supported. They may decline their body slightly by sitting propped up on cushions or a bench (known as 'inclined sitting'). Fold a small towel and place it behind their knee, making sure that the towel edge moves right into the knee crease (popliteal crease). Have them draw their thigh towards their chest and bend their knee, keeping the towel in place. They should then take hold of their shin and pull their heel in towards their buttock using the towel as a pivot. Have them hold the fully stretched position for 10–20 seconds and then release. They then straighten their knee completely, tightening their quadriceps muscles (knee brace, Exercise 8.1) and repeat.

### Variations
Have your client perform the exercise in a kneeling position, sitting back towards their heels. Greater overpressure is placed onto the joint so ensure that

they take their bodyweight through the hands placed on the floor. If they cannot reach the floor comfortably, use two blocks (yoga bricks) placed on the floor level with their hips, and have them place their hands on these.

### Points to note

The aim of this exercise is to gradually stretch the tightened tissues around the knee. These include the ligaments and joint capsule which may have been affected by swelling that has clotted to stiffen the tissues. It is important to allow the tissues to 'pay out' gradually, placing a small amount of stress on them over an extended period. It is common for the exercise to be uncomfortable but it should not be painful. In addition, the discomfort should ease over the period of the stretch. If pain is intense, or increases throughout the stretch, release the exercise and have them rest the knee until the pain has gone.

---

### Exercise 8.4 Short range quadriceps contraction

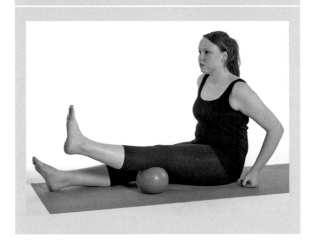

### Aims and usage

To work the quadriceps muscles within inner range only

### Starting position and instructions

Begin with your client sitting on the floor or a bench with their knee bent to 20 degrees. Place a 10–15cm rolled towel, medicine ball or block (soft yoga block) beneath their lower thigh for support. Have them tighten their thigh muscles (quadriceps contraction) and press the back of their thigh onto the block so that their heel lifts up. They continue lifting until their knee is locked out straight. Have them hold the locked position for 3–5 seconds and then lower under control.

### Variations

Vary the height of the block to give less movement range (lower block) or greater movement range (higher block).

### Points to note

The inner range action of the quadriceps emphasises the lower fibres of vastus medialis, which are positioned transversely (across the thighbone) compared to the other fibres that run longitudinally (in line with the thighbone). These are called the *vastus medialis obliquus* (VMO).

## Exercise 8.5 Quads re-strengthening using leg extension

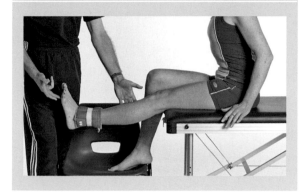

### Aims and usage

To re-strengthen the quadriceps muscles in a non-weight-bearing position

### Starting position and instructions

Begin with your client sitting on the edge of a gym bench or table with their foot resting on the floor. The bench should completely support their thigh, coming to just short of the back of the knee. Place a weight bag over their ankle and have them tighten their thigh (quadriceps) to straighten their knee. They should draw their toes towards them (dorsiflexion) and lock their knee completely, holding the fully locked position for 3–5 seconds before lowering under control.

### Variations

• Place a 2–5cm thick pad beneath their lower thigh to angle their thigh upwards. As they straighten their leg it reaches the point of maximum leverage when it is horizontal. By angling the thigh, maximum leverage occurs just short of full extension meaning that during the final degrees of extension the leverage is reducing,

effectively making the weight lighter to encourage full knee locking (*see* Figure 8.2).

• You may use a resistance band instead of a weight bag. To use a band, fix it beneath the bench and ensure that you take up any slack in the band when the knee is at rest so any effective resistance is applied throughout the movement range.

• This exercise may also be performed on a leg extension machine in the gym. This unit has an adjustable pad for different leg lengths, and a range of motion limiter to enable work on one part of the motion range alone (*see* multigym leg extension, Exercise 8.14).

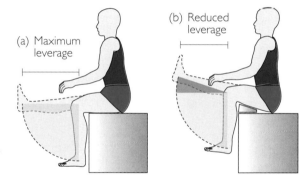

**Figure 8.2** Leverage effects during leg extension

### Points to note

This is a non-weight-bearing starting position meaning that the knee is subjected to less compression loading. If the foot is kept off the floor (bench higher so the heel clears the floor), slight traction is placed through the knee. Although this reduces joint loading further, contact with the floor allows the muscles to rest completely (known as a *relaxation stop*) between repetitions. This rest allows fresh blood to enter the working muscles, meaning that the muscles won't tire as easily.

## Exercise 8.6 Leg press using a ball

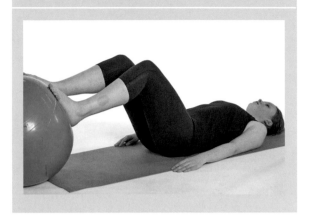

### Aims and usage

To work the leg muscles in closed chain format (*see* Chapter 3)

### Starting position and instructions

Begin with your client sitting on the floor, facing a wall. Place a gym ball (Swiss ball) between the wall and their foot so that their knee is bent (flexed) by 20–30 degrees. Have them press their foot into the ball, trying to straighten their leg. They should hold the point of maximum tension for 5–10 seconds and then release.

### Variations

Deflate the ball (softer) to provide less resistance and a greater motion range; inflate (harder) to offer greater resistance and less range.

### Points to note

• By adjusting your client's sitting distance from the ball you can change the range of motion at their knee. To practise knee locking, have them focus the movement on the final 10 degrees of extension.

### Definition

A relaxation stop is a point at which a limb is allowed to rest on the floor or supporting surface to allow muscles to relax between repetitions of an exercise. Where a relaxation stop is not provided muscles work under continuous tension.

• Ensure that your client's knee does not hyperextend. If the back of their knee has a tendency to drop back behind their leg line, place a block behind the knee to prevent this.

## Exercise 8.7 Leg press using a band

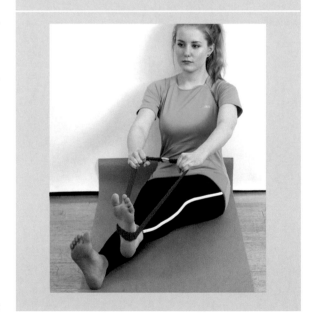

### Aims and usage

Closed chain leg muscle work

## Starting position and instructions

Begin with your client sitting with their back to a wall. Have them loop a resistance band around their foot and take up the slack so the band is tight with their knee bent. They should press their leg out straight against the resistance of the band and hold the locked position for 3–5 seconds before releasing.

## Variations

You can limit the client to part of the movement range, for example, taking the knee from 100 degrees flexion to 30, to work mid-range only, or 20 degrees flexion to full extension, to work end-range. This can be useful following surgery where the patient's surgeon may instruct that you avoid certain movement ranges during rehab.

## Points to note

• Make sure your client turns their head away from the band in case it slips off their foot.

• The client may also use this action as a combined strength and stretch action to perform an active knee extension (AKE) exercise. For this movement, have them begin lying on their back, loop the band around their foot and ask them to press out straight. Bringing their foot closer to their body increases hamstrings stretch while taking it away reduces the stretch.

## Clinical scenario – knee swelling

In the acute stage of healing it is important not to perform exercise therapy which would disrupt the healing tissues. Initial management is by the protect, rest, ice, compression and elevation (PRICE) method. Cold and compression around the knee should be used with the leg rested in an elevated position (foot on a stool when sitting) to limit the spread of swelling. Where swelling is pronounced and older, steeper elevation is useful and you may wish to modify the hamstrings stretch supported by doorframe (Exercise 7.10). The position is held with both legs against a wall (legs straight but relaxed) for 15–20 minutes to allow knee swelling to drain through the pull of gravity. To encourage lymph flow back through the body the hips may be elevated by 10–15cm on cushions or yoga blocks. Once the swelling begins to subside (3–5 days post injury), start with the knee brace (Exercise 8.1) to encourage quadriceps work and limit muscle wasting, followed by the straight leg raise (Exercise 8.2) to ensure that the quadriceps are able to fully lock the knee. Use short range quadriceps contractions (Exercise 8.4) followed by leg extension to re-strengthen the quads in cases where muscle wasting or pain inhibition has occurred. In the latter case the use of tactile cueing is important with a trainer touching/stimulating the muscle to encourage a full force contraction.

The above exercises have the advantage that they are non-weight-bearing, meaning that they won't load the knee joint. However, their disadvantage is that they are not fully functional in that they work one muscle group (quadriceps) in isolation from others (hamstrings and hip musculature). When the knee locking is possible use leg press using a ball (Exercise 8.6) and leg press using a band (Exercise 8.7) to work the knee and hip musculature together in a partial weight-bearing (closed chain) position.

## Exercise 8.8 Step-up

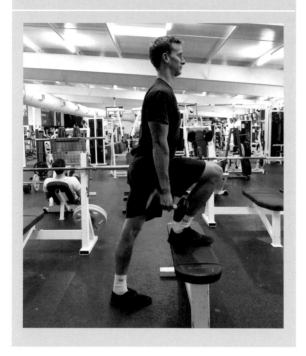

### Aims and usage

To re-strengthen the leg musculature in a functional step action

### Starting position and instructions

Begin with your client standing in front of a bench or step. Have them place the injured (for example, right) foot onto the bench with the foot correctly aligned (facing forwards and slightly turned out). Next, have them step onto the bench with their left leg and then off again with the same leg. They should perform 5 reps and then swap to place the left foot on the bench and step with their right, again for 5 reps.

### Variations

• Step up and down with both legs rather than leaving one on the step. This action demands accurate foot placement with each step rather than at the beginning of each set only.

• Step onto the bench with their uninjured (left) leg and then down leading with their left leg. In this way the injured (right) leg only performs eccentric activity rather than concentric, a useful technique where muscle strength is poor and concentric activity is limited. Use sticks or crutches to lighten the body load further.

• Increase the bench height to increase the workload on the quadriceps muscles.

### Points to note

Make sure that the bench or step is stable. Gym benches may be placed against a wall, while commercial step benches have rubber feet to guard against slipping. Do not have your client step onto a padded (upholstered) gym bench as the vinyl surface is unstable and the foot is liable to slip.

## Exercise 8.9 Step down from block

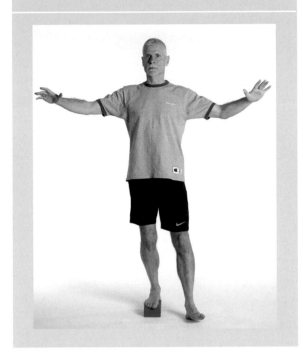

### Aims and usage
Eccentric muscle action emphasising knee-foot alignment

### Starting position and instructions
Begin with your client standing on a block, stool or step bench. Have them keep their injured (right) foot on the block and step down with their uninjured (left) foot. Ensure that the knee of their right foot stays over the outside of their foot so that they take the weight towards the outer (lateral) side of their foot. Make sure they do not flatten the foot and/or allow their knee to move inwards to a 'knock knee' position.

### Variations
Begin with your client standing on a low step (a firm book is ideal) and build up the height to a small and then larger step. Home exercise clients can use a bottom step of a staircase, for example.

### Points to note
Make sure that the client maintains pelvic alignment, avoiding any tipping or dipping of the pelvis to the side. To cue the hip action focus on sucking the hip bone (greater trochanter) inwards to create a shallow hollow over the outside of the hip.

## Exercise 8.10 In-place carioca

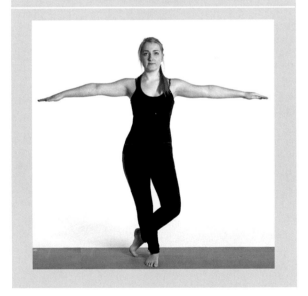

### Aims and usage
To apply multidirectional stress over the knee

### Starting position and instructions
Begin with your client standing in the centre of a room or corridor, facing the wall, with their

feet shoulder-width apart. Have them stand on their right foot and step behind it with their left foot, then they move their left foot back to the starting position and step in front of their right.

## Variations

• Have your client bend their knees further as their foot touches the floor to produce a combined step-dip action with the leg to increase muscle work.
• Have them jump slightly on each step to increase joint loading and movement speed.
• Ask them to perform a moving carioca by sidestepping to the right as they step in front and behind their right leg and then return, sidestepping to the left as they step in front and behind their left leg.

## Points to note

Both legs work in this action and the coordination and balance is quite challenging. With the right foot on the ground the stepping action of the left imparts flexion and rotation stress to the right knee. This is a useful action to progress from single plane actions, such as leg extension, before returning to sport. The action may also be used as part of a functional test battery to assess fitness to play following knee injury.

---

## Exercise 8.11 Balance board knee dip

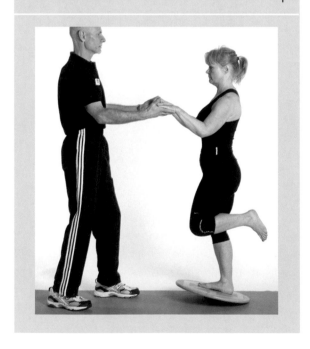

## Aims and usage

To improve proprioception and stabilisation of the knee on a mobile surface

## Starting position and instructions

Begin with your client facing a wall or wallbar with their right (injured) foot in the centre of a balance board. Begin with their knee locked out straight and then ask them to unlock it by bending it to 10 degrees and then lock it out straight again. Have them perform 10 reps of this action, keeping their pelvis aligned (do not allow them to dip their pelvis or their hip to sag outwards).

## Variations

• Have your client perform the action initially with their hands on the wall, then move their hands away from the wall but keep them outstretched to the side to assist balance. Finally, have them drop their hands to their sides to remove balance assistance and rely on balance sensations (proprioception) coming from their leg alone.

• Have them perform the same action using a vibrating platform (vibration exercise or VbX). The effect is to increase limb circulation and muscle condition as well as improve balance. VbX was originally introduced in Russia in the 1970s to maintain the physical condition of cosmonauts. The technique has been researched extensively by the European Space Agency (ESA) and is used regularly within physiotherapy (*see* Cochrane 2011 for review).

### Points to note

You can get balance boards in several different types (*see* Figure 4.5). A rocker board has a semi-circular block which restricts movement to one plane only (known as 'uniplanar motion'). Placing the block in a forwards-backwards direction allows flexion and extension, while placing it in a side-to-side direction allows abduction and adduction (*see* Figure 4.5a). A balance board has a dome-shaped block which allows movement in all directions (multiplanar motion) and so is more challenging to balance (*see* Figure 4.5b).

## Exercise 8.12 Balance board throw and catch

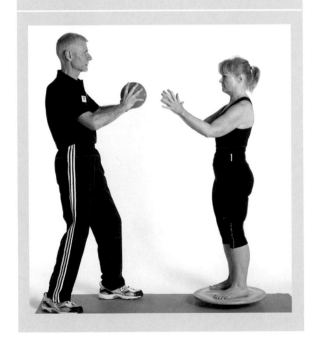

### Aims and usage

To improve knee stability on a mobile surface.

### Starting position and instructions

Begin with your client standing on a balance board (wobble board) with their feet hip-width apart, 1–1.5m from a wall. Have them hold a ball in both hands and throw and catch the ball, bouncing it off the wall. Advise them to keep their knees slightly flexed ('soft') rather than locked out to allow them to vary their body position more easily.

### Variations

Have your client stand on one leg with their weight-bearing foot placed in the centre of the balance board.

### Points to note

By focusing on throwing and catching the ball, two things happen:

• The momentum of the ball induces forces in the knee which tend to displace it, meaning that the knee-stabilising muscles have to work harder.

• Your client's attention is taken from the knee to the ball, making the stabilisation of the knee more automatic (less conscious), emphasising the autonomous stage of motor learning.

### Exercise 8.13 Single leg band resisted throw and catch

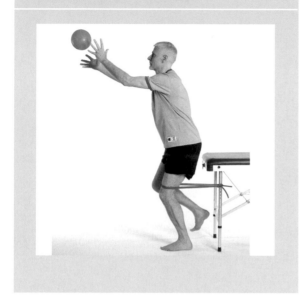

• Throwing the ball forwards provides flexion-extension directed (sagittal motion) stress on the knee while throwing to the side provides abduction-adduction directed (frontal motion) stress.

## Points to note

The resistance band is only used to introduce a pulling/angular (shear) stress to the knee. Do not use a band which is so strong that the client has to work hard to prevent it pulling them towards the wallbar.

### Exercise 8.14 Multigym leg extension

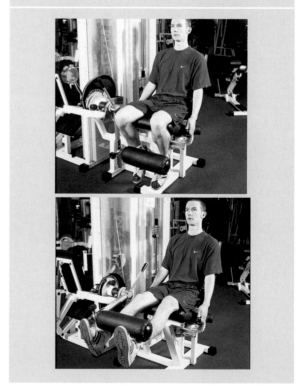

## Aims and usage

To work knee stability in a functional floor-standing position

## Starting position and instructions

Begin with your client standing on their injured (left) leg with a resistance band looped around their thigh and attached to a wallbar or machine upright. Have them move back slightly so the band is comfortably tight, but not pulling them off balance. Stand in front of them holding a standard ball (football, basketball) or medicine ball. Throw and catch the ball to your client while they maintain their single leg balance position.

## Variations

• Using a medicine ball rather than an unweighted ball increases the workload because the momentum of the ball provides a greater challenge to balance.

## Aims and usage

To re-strengthen the quadriceps muscles in a non-weight-bearing position

## Starting position and instructions

Begin by adjusting the machine seat and shin pad for comfort. Align the machine pivot to the centre of the outside of your client's knee (lateral joint line). Have them straighten their legs, making sure that they lock their knees out fully. Ask them to pause in the straight position and then lower under control.

## Variations

• Have your client lift with one leg at a time, adjusting the machine resistance to allow for differences between their injured and uninjured sides.

• Lift with both legs and lower with just their injured leg to focus on the eccentric phase of movement.

• Some machines on the rehabilitation market have an in-built range limiter. This allows you to restrict movement to one part of the range only, which can be useful following certain types of knee surgery (*see* Figure 8.3).

## Points to note

Having your client draw their toes towards them (foot dorsiflexion) mimics the leg position at heel strike during walking and running and can make contracting the quadriceps muscles easier.

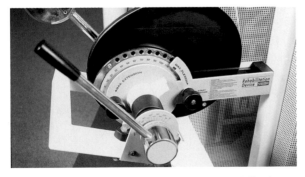

**Figure 8.3** Certain machines on the rehabilitation market have an in-built limiter.

## Clinical scenario – medial collateral ligament (MCL) tear

Rehabilitation following a medial collateral ligament (MCL) injury on the inside of the knee initially has similarities to that of the knee swelling scenario and that of osteoarthrosis (OA). Where inflammation is present, use the PRICE treatment and where the knee has been stiff for a prolonged period, capsular stretching can be helpful. As movement and strength is regained, more varied stress is then required to prepare the knee for work or sport. Twisting and side-to-side actions and rapid movements are all required as the knee will be subjected to these at some time and must be prepared to meet the challenge. Progress from step up/down (Exercise 8.8 and 8.9) actions to in-place carioca (Exercise 8.10). Have your client perform this slowly to begin with, as it places both side-to-side (valgus) and twisting (torsion) stress on the knee which stress the ligament. By keeping the injured leg still and moving the unaffected leg, the knee joint on the injured side is stressed to encourage both knee stability through muscle action and ligament strength. Use the balance board knee dip (Exercise 8.11) and balance board throw and catch (Exercise 8.12) to encourage further muscular stability and enhance joint sense (proprioception), which is impaired due to ligament injury. Strength may be built up further using the free weight squat (Exercise 8.15) in the gym and the overhead squat (Exercise 8.16) to introduce further balance work. Plyometric exercises including the box jump (Exercise 8.19) and hurdle jump (Exercise 8.20) again challenge knee stability and introduce speed and muscle reaction time.

## Exercise 8.15 Free weight squat

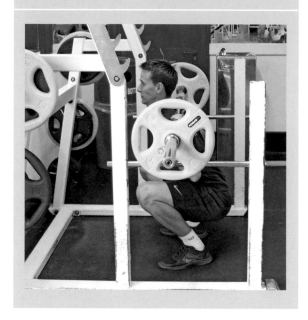

### Aims and usage

To work the leg and low back musculature and teach correct lumbopelvic and lower limb alignment during a squat action

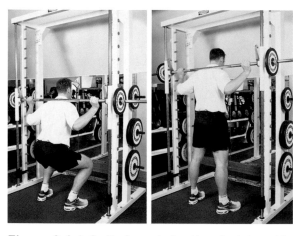

**Figure 8.4** A Smith frame helps the client to guide and support the barbell with proper technique.

### Starting position and instructions

Begin with your client standing with their feet hip-width apart and turned out slightly. If they are new to squatting have them stand in front of a gym bench to act as a relaxation stop. Ask them to bend their knees ensuring that their knee passes over their foot and their trunk remains upright. They should then straighten their knees again, maintaining good alignment as they come up.

### Variations

• Where your client's legs are quite weak, use a gym bench for support in the low position. Advise them to touch their buttocks to the bench but not to sit down completely.

• If your client has problems keeping their trunk upright, have them begin facing a wall to use their fingertips on the wall to monitor their upper body position.

• If their calf/Achilles is tight, get them to raise their heels on a small block to reduce the amount of ankle bending (dorsiflexion) as they descend.

• To progress to a weighted squat (Exercise 8.16), use a wooden pole across your client's shoulders in lieu of a barbell to begin with. This ensures that the client masters correct technique before resistance is added. Using a frame to guide and support the barbell (Smith frame) protects against poor technique, which could endanger the low back especially (*see* Figure 8.4).

### Points to note

• As your client bends their knee it should pass over the centre of their foot. A knock knee (genu valgum) position flattens the foot, and stresses the inner knee. A bow legged position (genu varum) places the bodyweight onto the outer edge of the foot, and stresses the outer knee. Both positions should be corrected by reducing the depth of the squat and focusing on knee alignment.

• Initially the depth of the squat should be limited, stopping when the hips reach the horizontal position. With practice, your client should deepen the squat by taking the hips below the horizontal position. Where a full squat is performed (buttocks to calf) the action must be slow and controlled with precise alignment. The full squat can be useful in sports which may require this degree of loaded knee motion such as street dance, gymnastics and some martial arts. However, this variation should be practised initially under the supervision of an experienced personal trainer.

## Exercise 8.16 Overhead squat

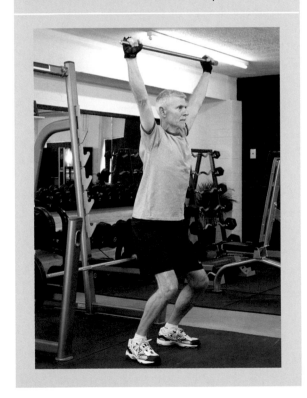

### Aims and usage
To work the leg and trunk musculature for strength and stability

### Starting position and instructions
Have your client grasp a light bar (a broom handle is fine to begin with) in both hands and reach it overhead. Ensure they keep their elbows locked and their chest lifted (thoracic spine extension). Have them draw the exercise bar back so that their arms are positioned level with or slightly behind their ears. They should maintain this arm position as they perform a squat action, pausing in the lower position with their thighs horizontal. They press their legs out straight to stand back up.

### Variations
• Use a towel or rope held in each hand instead of a bar.
• To increase motion range, your client should allow their buttocks to lower below the horizontal position. However, ensure that they keep their chest lifted and do not allow it to drop causing their upper back (thoracic spine) to round.

### Points to note
To begin, have your client rehearse the free weight squat (Exercise 8.15), ensuring that they have optimal lower limb alignment throughout.

## Exercise 8.17 Deadlift

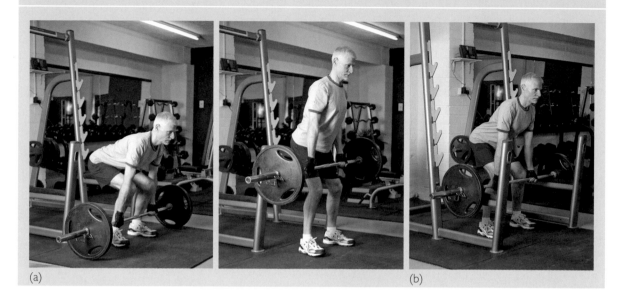

(a)  (b)

### Aims and usage

To strengthen the legs and trunk in a functional lifting action

### Starting position and instructions

Begin with your client standing in front of a barbell. Have them place their feet hip-width apart with feet facing forwards but turned out 10–15 degrees. The barbell should just touch their shins. They should then bend their knees to squat down, keeping their back aligned with a slight hollow in the low back (neutral lumbar lordosis), their chest open (thoracic spine extension) and their shoulders drawn back (scapular retraction). Ask them to grip the bar with their knuckles up (overgrasp) and lightly draw their abdominal muscles inwards to brace their trunk. They should then push with their legs to straighten their knees and lift the bar, keeping it close to their body, before lowering using the same precise alignment.

### Variations

• If your client has not deadlifted before, begin with the weight lifted on blocks to reduce the depth of the squat (b). The lower position should bend the knees to a maximum of 90 degrees (partial deadlift).

• Have them perform a dumbbell deadlift by holding a dumbbell in each hand and taking them to the side of their legs as they squat down. This action keeps the weight close to their bodyline.

### Points to note

• The aim of this action is for the client to keep the bar close to their body. If the bar creeps forwards of their bodyline, the leverage effect is increased. The leverage effect multiplies the weight making the bar in effect heavier. This often occurs at the mid-point of the movement and can cause the spine to bend (flex), greatly increasing stress on the back.

• The complexities of this exercise are such that close supervision by a personal trainer is warranted. Ensuring the correct technique is learnt from the very start avoids the need to correct faults that can develop when lifting heavier weights.

## Exercise 8.18 Lunge

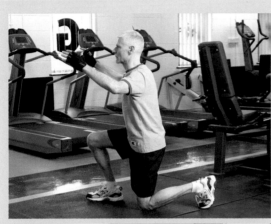

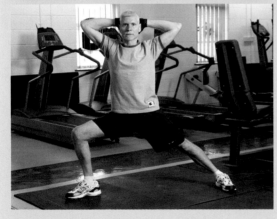

### Starting position and instructions

Begin with your client standing with their feet shoulder-width apart. Ask them to step forwards with their right leg to a distance of about half the length of their leg (half leg length). Have them bend their knees, lowering their left knee to the ground and keeping their right over their right (leading) foot. Keeping their body upright, they should look forwards before pressing back up to the standing position and repeating the action, leading with their left leg.

### Variations

• Increase the range of motion by having your client step further forwards so that the trailing hip is moved further into extension.

• Reduce the stepping distance (quarter leg length or less) so that the action is more directly downwards than forwards. This reduces work on the thigh muscles (quadriceps) and proportionally increases it on the buttock muscles (gluteals).

• Have them perform a side lunge by stepping forwards and to the side ('little toe' side). This action changes the loading on both knees by combining forward-backward (sagittal) motion forces with side to side (frontal) forces.

### Aims and usage

To work the legs and trunk in a functional lunge action

### Points to note

• In the classic free-standing lunge, the trailing leg knee should touch the floor level with the heel of the leading leg. The gap between the two should be approximately the same as the gap between the feet at the start of the exercise.

## Exercise 8.19 Box jump

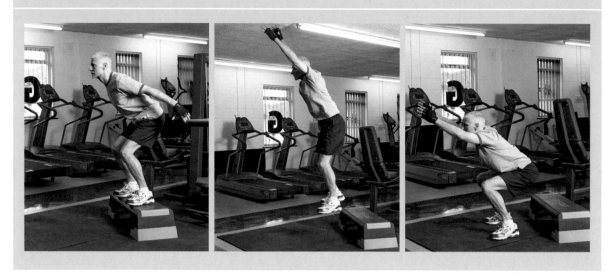

### Aims and usage

To introduce jumping stress on the leg in a controlled manner

### Starting position and instructions

Begin with your client standing on a gym bench or box (step bench) positioned securely. Have them stand with their feet shoulder-width apart and feet facing forwards. They should extend their arms forwards or sideways to assist with their balance. Then, ask them to jump down from the box, bending their knees as they do so to soften the landing impact. They then turn around and step back onto the bench, readjust their posture and repeat.

### Variations

• Making the box higher increases training intensity while making it lower reduces it.

• Once they have landed and bent their knees (squat landing), have them jump back up vertically so that their feet leave the ground, or jump forwards and upwards.

• Using a low bench, have them jump off sideways to introduce side facing (frontal) forces to the knee.

• Increase intensity and joint loading by having them perform the exercise on a single leg.

### Points to note

• This action is a plyometric exercise which works for muscle strength and recoil of elastic structures within the muscle. It is known as a 'depth drop' in plyometrics, and when followed by jumping back up from the squat landing position it is a 'depth jump'.

## Exercise 8.20 Hurdle jump

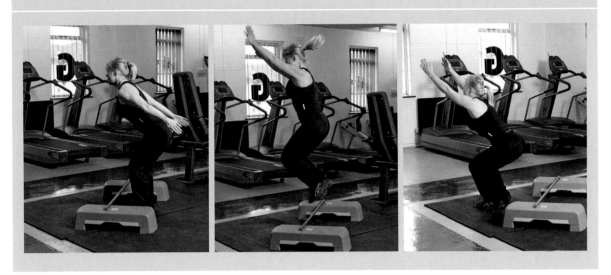

### Aims and usage

To introduce controlled shearing stress to the knee

### Starting position and instructions

Stand your client side-on to a line on the floor or low height hurdle (stick balanced on two small blocks). Have them keep their feet hip-width apart and bend their knees, reaching their arms out to the side for balance. Ask them to jump across the line/hurdle, bending their knees to absorb shock as they land. They then jump back and repeat the action.

### Variations

• Increasing the height of the hurdle and not jumping as far sideways increases leg muscle work and compression (downward) stress, but reduces shearing (crossways) stress and joint demands on the knee.

• Performing the exercise single legged increases stability and balance demands.

• Performing the exercise while twisting the body (jump and turn 90 degrees) introduces torsional (twisting) forces on the knee.

### Points to note

Following injury it is common to use well controlled actions which serve to protect the knee. Although this is correct, as it protects the knee, in the later stages of rehab prior to returning to sport or work it is necessary to challenge the knee in a less protected way to build reaction speed, joint stability and predictive ability. This exercise is useful to provide a bridge between controlled training exercise and less controlled competitive sport.

## Definition

A *plyometric* exercise (also called shock exercise) combines concentric and eccentric muscle work with no rest between the two actions. Muscle force is produced by *contraction* of the muscle fibre mechanism (actin-myosin coupling) and elastic *recoil* of the connective tissue framework surrounding the fibres (endomysium, epimysium) and the muscle tendon. Plyometrics are used to build speed and power for sport.

### Exercise 8.21 Standing static cycle

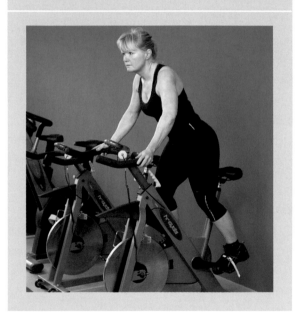

### Aims and usage

To develop leg power and endurance

### Starting position and instructions

Begin with your client sitting on a static cycle, using the toe straps if available. Adjust the resistance so that it is quite high. Have them take their weight on the handlebars and stand up on the pedals. They then cycle in a standing position for 10–15 seconds and then sit back onto the saddle and reduce the resistance to recover. Have them do 5 reps.

### Variations

• Reduce the resistance to allow your client to cycle faster, working for speed rather than power.
• Have them take more weight onto their arms (lean forwards) to reduce knee joint loading.

### Points to note

If you have the resistance set too low, the pedals may spin quickly as your client stands on them, making him/her unstable. Increasing the resistance makes the pedals more stable to stand on, and once pedalling you may reduce the resistance to suit your client's ability.

## Clinical scenario – knee osteoarthrosis (OA)

Arthrosis is a degenerative condition of the bone surfaces within the knee. The bone condition is the primary effect, but secondary effects of joint stiffness and muscle wasting are often more important to day-to-day function. In an acute flare-up of arthritis, where inflammation is marked, treatment is as for the knee swelling clinical scenario (see page 101). Once inflammation has reduced and the knee is no longer hot and swollen, capsular stretching and muscle strengthening is important. The quadriceps (rectus femoris) stretch in standing (Exercise 7.11) may be usefully modified as a capsular stretch. Begin by asking your client to allow their knee to move forwards of the body and out slightly (hip flexion and abduction) and then to draw their heel in towards their buttock very gradually, allowing time for the knee to stretch. Once the maximum knee stretch is achieved, they should maintain the knee angle and pull the whole thigh back and in (hip extension and adduction), trying to bring both knees together.

To increase the intensity of the joint stretch use the capsular stretch to knee (Exercise 8.3). Ask the client to allow their knee to ease gradually, holding the exercise for 20–30 seconds without increasing the intensity of the pull on their shin. Expect it to take 2–3 weeks for the knee stiffness to fully release.

In parallel to the joint stretching use a progressive re-strengthening programme. Begin with non-weight bearing exercises such as short range quadriceps contraction (Exercise 8.4) and quads re-strengthening using leg extension (Exercise 8.5) and move on to leg press using a ball (Exercise 8.6) and leg press using a band (Exercise 8.7). Once strength begins to return, step up (Exercise 8.8) and step down from block (Exercise 8.9) can make tackling stairs easier and increase quadriceps strength still further. Even where the knee arthritis is quite bad, providing the joint is not inflamed it is still possible to strengthen the supporting knee muscles.

# SHIN, ANKLE AND FOOT

# 9

## ANATOMY REFRESHER

### SHIN

The shin consists of two bones, the tibia, or shin bone proper, on the inside and the fibula, or splint bone, on the outside. On top of these are the long shin and calf muscles which are arranged in groups separated by membranes (fascia) (*see* Figure 9.1).

On the front and outside of the shin (anterolateral) is the thick tibialis anterior muscle which pulls the foot upwards, and beneath it the toe extensor muscles (extensor digitorum longus and extensor hallucis longus, usually shortened to EDL and EHL). This group of muscles represents the anterior compartment and is a common area for shin splints, giving a dull ache along the outside of the shin after running or jumping activities. To the side of the fibula bone are the peroneus muscles (peroneus longus and peroneus tertius). These swing the ankle outwards and support the outside of the ankle joint, making them important to restrengthen following ankle sprains.

On the back of the leg we have the calf, which actually consists of both a long and short muscle. They both work over the ankle, but the long one (gastrocnemius) goes above the knee

and the short one (soleus) below. This fact is important when stretching, because the long calf muscle is more effectively stretched with the knee locked out straight, the short muscle with the knee allowed to bend.

Beneath the calf muscles are the toes' bending (flexor) muscles, flexor digitorum longus (FDL) and flexor hallucis longus (FHL), and the tibialis posterior, which is the main inverter of the foot

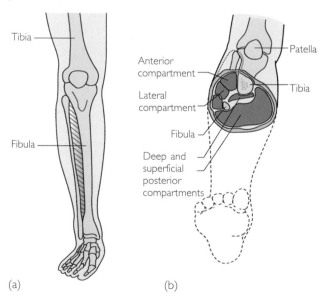

(a)    (b)

**Figure 9.1** The shin fascia

(turns the sole of the foot inwards). The tibialis anterior and posterior are both important muscles which support the bodyweight on the ankle when standing on one leg and are often worked in ankle stabilising programmes after ligament injury or fractures of the lower leg and ankle.

The calf muscles attach into the heel bone (calcaneus) via the strong Achilles tendon. This is the largest tendon in the body, measuring on average about 15cm long and 2cm thick. It is so strong that laboratory experiments have shown it to be capable of withstanding loads of up to 17 times bodyweight. The Achilles joins the two large calf muscles (gastrocnemius and soleus) to the heel bone and transmits the power of the calf into the foot to allow you to push off against the ground during walking and running. The tendon passes across the back of the heel where it is separated from the bone by a balloon-like structure, the Achilles bursa. The Achilles is highly elastic, a function which is increased by the fact that the tendon twists through 90 degrees throughout its length, and unwinds as it is stretched. Each end of the tendon has a good blood supply, but in the central portion the blood flow is not as good, and for this reason ruptures (tendon snapping) often occur at this point. One of the most common conditions affecting the Achilles is tendon pain (known as 'tendinopathy'), which normally begins as a dull tendon ache after running.

The calf muscles themselves may tear during explosive actions such as lunging for a ball in tennis, and it is important to identify which muscle and which part of the muscle is affected to develop an accurate rehab programme.

## ANKLE AND FOOT

The ankle joint is formed between the bottom of the shin bones and the rear foot bones. You

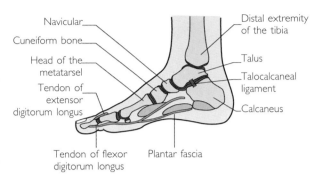

**Figure 9.2** The ankle joint

actually have two rear foot bones: the heel (calcaneus) and ankle bone itself on top (talus). The ankle bone sits like a square mortise within the two shin bones (*see* Figure 9.2).

As you point your foot downwards and upwards the ankle bone slides between the shin bones. It is held in place by two sets of ligaments: on the inside of the ankle is the medial ligament, and on the outside the lateral ligament. Closer inspection of the lateral ligament shows it to be made up of three bands, the front one pointing forwards, the middle band pointing to the floor and the rear band pointing backwards. When you sprain your ankle, it is the front band of the lateral ligament which is most commonly injured. This portion will be stressed by an exercise that combines ankle pointing (plantarflexion) with turning the sole inwards (inversion), an important consideration when designing rehab programmes following ankle sprain.

The sole of the foot forms two main arches (*see* Figure 9.3). On the inside is the medial longitudinal arch. The top of the arch is the navicular bone, and the distance of this bone to the floor is often used as a measure of arch

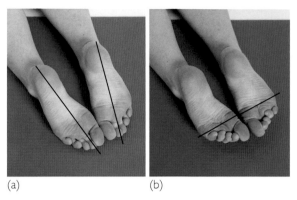

**Figure 9.3** The two main arches of the foot: (a) the medial longitudinal arch and (b) the transverse arch

height. Across the centre of the foot is the transverse arch which forms a shallow dip between the ball of the foot (first metatarsal phalangeal joint) and the fourth and fifth toes. As weight is taken onto the foot, the arches flatten and give the foot its natural spring. The arches are maintained by muscle action, and through the strength and elasticity of the foot ligaments and plantarfascia (plantar aponeurosis). This later structure is a dense, triangular, fibrous structure stretching from the inner front of the heel bone (medial calcaneal tuberosity) to the base of the toe knuckles (metatarsal heads). The plantarfascia is tightened or 'wound up' by flexing the toes (known as the 'Windlass effect') and the medial arch raises as a result.

The muscles of the sole of the foot should be strong to support the arches and take strain away from the other foot structures. The popularity of wearing training shoes, however, allows the foot muscles to weaken. As a result, foot strengthening exercises involving barefoot actions are often used to re-strengthen the foot after injury and foot arch pain.

**Exercise 9.1** Foot shortening

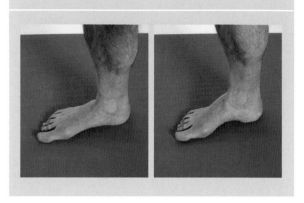

### Aims and usage
To strengthen the foot arch muscles

### Starting position and instructions
Begin with your client sitting with their bare foot flat on the floor, knee directly above their ankle. Have them press their knee over the outside of their ankle and at the same time draw the ball of their foot (big toe side) backwards towards their heel. They should hold the high arch position for 5–10 seconds and then release.

### Variations
• Have your client place load through their foot by leaning their trunk forwards and pressing down onto their knee. Have them perform the exercise in standing and/or single leg standing to further increase weight-bearing.

### Points to note
Make sure that your client does not curl their toes and simply dig them into the ground. The action is to raise the arch (medial longitudinal arch) rather than flex the toes.

## Exercise 9.2 Toe spread

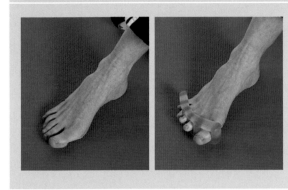

### Aims and usage
To restore active toe spreading (abduction)

### Starting position and instructions
Begin with your client sitting barefoot, their heel resting on the floor. Get them to focus their attention on their toes and try to spread them out to the side away from the centre of their foot. Have them hold the spread position for 3–5 seconds and then release.

### Variations
• Have them place their foot flat on the floor. They should then gently pull their toes apart (passive movement) and press their foot into the floor, attempting the hold the spread-toe position.
• Use a commercial toe spreader (*see* photo) or place small foam blocks between their toes to stretch the interossei muscles (between the metatarsal bones on toes 2–4) for 3–5 minutes prior to trying the toe spread action.
• Have them practise barefoot sports such as yoga and use barefoot shoes to encourage natural toe spread during other activities.

### Points to note
• Toe spreading is a natural function of the foot that is lost when we wear tight fitting shoes. At forefoot contact, toe spread enhances the gripping action of the foot. When your client has tried this exercise for some time and/or begun to walk in bare feet or practise barefoot sports such as yoga, it is common for their forefoot to broaden.
• This action is performed by the abductor hallucis (big toe), abductor digiti minimi (little toe) and dorsal interossei (toes 2–4) muscles.

## Exercise 9.3 Active inversion and eversion

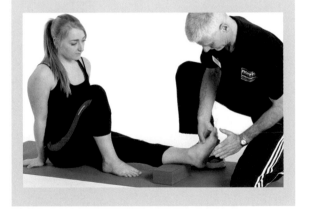

### Aims and usage
To re-strengthen the ankle inversion (tibialis anterior and posterior) and eversion (peronei) muscles

### Starting position and instructions
Begin with your client sitting on the floor barefoot with their left (injured) leg placed on a block so the heel clears the floor. Have them keep their kneecap pointing to the ceiling (they should not rotate their leg at the hip) and turn their foot

so the sole faces inwards (inversion) and then outwards (eversion).

## Variations

• Have your client cross their injured leg over their uninjured leg at the shin, and perform the action sitting on a chair or gym bench.

• Have them perform the action weight-bearing in sitting (partial weight-bearing) or standing (full weight-bearing). The action is now to lift the inner and then outer edge of their foot off the floor.

## Points to note

The open chain position (foot off the floor) is easier to learn initially, but the closed chain position (foot on the floor) is more functional. Your client should progress to closed chain and build holding time from 3–5 seconds to 10–15 seconds.

---

### Exercise 9.4 Balance board

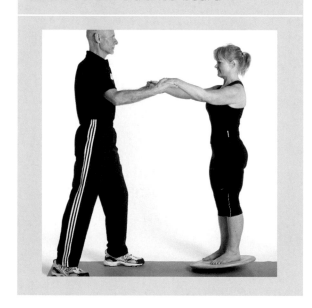

Have them rock the board from side to side, trying to stop at the mid-point with neither edge of the board touching the ground. Use the same action forward and back, again asking them to stop at the mid-point so the board is balancing on its centre dome alone. Build the holding time from 10–20 seconds up to 2 minutes, with the aim that your client stays on the board dome but avoids the edges touching the floor.

## Variations

• Have your client perform the exercise with their eyes closed. Taking the visual cue away increases the reliance on proprioceptive information coming from the joints.

• Have them stand on one leg rather than both, placing their single foot in the centre of the board, directly over the dome.

• Have them stand in front of the board and place their injured (right) foot onto the centre before transferring their weight onto and off the board, keeping their left toes just on the floor for balance.

## Aims and usage

To work stability and muscle reaction time of the ankle musculature on an unstable base

## Starting position and instructions

Begin with your client standing on a balance (wobble) board facing a wall. Initially, they should use their hands on the wall for balance, but release one hand and then both as their balance improves.

## Points to note

Also see balance board knee dip (Exercise 8.11) for information about this type of exercise, and the difference between rocker and balance boards.

## Exercise 9.5 Ankle stability using standing body twist

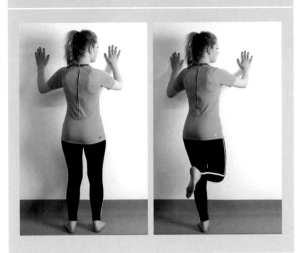

### Aims and usage

To work stability and muscle reaction time of the ankle musculature on a stable base

### Starting position and instructions

Begin with your client standing on their injured leg, in bare feet, facing a wall. Have them place their hands on the wall for support, and as their skill improves encourage them to release first one and then both hands. They should slightly flex (soften) their knee and turn their trunk from side to side, while maintaining their balance by gripping the floor with their foot.

### Variations

• Have your client begin by standing still until their balance improves. They should aim to stand for 5–10 seconds, progressing to 20–30 seconds.
• Use a weight shift (side-to-side) action prior to trunk rotation.
• Have them keep their head forwards, fixing their eyes on a single spot, and progress to them moving their head with their trunk.

### Points to note

If your client locks their knee out stiffly, the rotation force (torsion) on the knee is increased and the collateral ligaments are placed under greater stress.

### Clinical scenario – ankle sprain

Ankle sprain more commonly occurs to the outer (lateral) ligament with associated problems to the peroneal muscles running down the outside of the shin. Initially the aim is to limit swelling as this tends to build up quickly around the outer ankle bone (lateral malleolus). Gentle active inversion and eversion (Exercise 9.3) is used to encourage reabsorption of swelling and to stop the swelling from pooling. Performing the exercise in sitting begins the process of taking weight through the ankle, and depending on the severity of injury, you may walk with your ankle supported with a tape or brace. As strength increases it is important to use unstable surfaces and the balance board (Exercise 9.4) is the best choice here. This may be used in sitting or standing, your client holding onto something to take some of their bodyweight (partial weight-bearing). Ankle stability using standing body twist (see Exercise 9.8, variations) provides the transition from partial to full weight-bearing. Once strength and stability has increased and your client is able to walk and jog lightly, use the hop and hold exercise (see Exercise 9.8, variations) to begin rapid actions. Varying from forwards-backwards to side-to-side and twisting actions introduces varying stresses to the ankle to facilitate multidirectional stability.

## Exercise 9.6 Straight leg heel raise

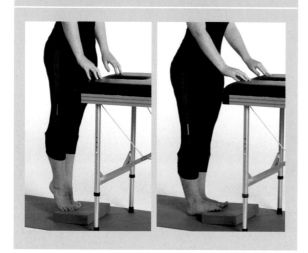

### Aims and usage

To strengthen the calf musculature

### Starting position and instructions

Begin with your client standing close to a wall or piece of machinery for support. Have them place the balls of their feet on a block or small step. They should allow their heels to lower below the level of their toes and then raise them again to lift them above the level of their toes. Have them remain in the raised position for 3–5 seconds before lowering.

### Variations

• Have your client perform the exercise on one leg (single heel raise), bending the knee of the opposite leg to fold the leg out of the way.
• Have them hold a dumbbell in one hand to increase workload.
• Emphasise the eccentric component of the movement by having them raise on both legs, and lower on just one.

### Points to note

• Keeping the knees locked out straight works the two major calf muscles: gastrocnemius (superficial), which attaches above the knee, and soleus (deep), which attaches below. Allowing the knee to bend slightly reduces tension in the gastrocnemius muscle and throws increased emphasis on the soleus.
• As well as strengthening the calf, stress is imposed on the Achilles tendon. High amounts of stress have been shown to stimulate useful remodelling of the Achilles tissue in cases of tendinopathy.

## Exercise 9.7 Bent knee heel raise

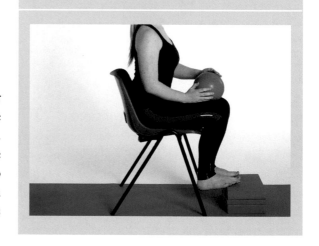

### Aims and usage

To strengthen the deep calf musculature

### Starting position and instructions

Begin with your client sitting with the balls of their feet raised on a block or step. Their knees should be bent to 90 degrees so that their shins are vertical. A weight (weight bag, medicine ball or barbell) may be placed on the lower thigh for resistance.

Have them allow their heels to lower below the level of their toes and then raise them to lift above the level of their toes again. They should remain in the raised position for 3–5 seconds before lowering.

## Variations

• Emphasise the eccentric component of the movement by having your client raise on both legs, and lower on just one.

• Increase the muscle overload by having them perform the action more slowly (superslow technique), taking 20–30 seconds for a single repetition rather than 3–5 seconds.

## Points to note

• The main emphasis of this exercise is on the soleus muscles as the gastrocnemius muscle attaches above the knee, so by bending the knee the latter muscle is relaxed.

• The tibialis posterior muscle (deep to soleus) also contributes to heel raising (plantarflexion). Although it produces significantly less power than the soleus or gastrocnemius it can still plantarflex the foot in cases where the Achilles tendon is ruptured. This is because the tibialis posterior attaches to the navicular bone of the foot rather than to the Achilles tendon.

### Exercise 9.8 Hop and hold

## Aims and usage

To build strength and power in the calf

## Starting position and instructions

Begin with your client standing in the centre of a clear floor. Have them stand on their right (recovering) leg and hop forwards, flexing their knee as they land. They should hold the position, remaining on one leg, and then hop again. Have them perform 5–10 repetitions before placing the other leg on the ground and resting.

## Variations

• As your client hops, have them twist their body 45 degrees to one side to land with their foot turned outwards. They should hop again, twisting their body 45 degrees to the other direction, landing with their foot turned inwards. Ensure they hold the movement at each landing.

• Have them hop from side to side, and then sideways in a line for five steps before returning for five steps. Ensure they hold the movement at each landing.

## Points to note

Holding the position on landing focuses on the balance component of the action. To build endurance and speed, do not have them hold the position, but instead use a continuous hopping action.

## Exercise 9.9 Anterior tibial stretch, kneeling

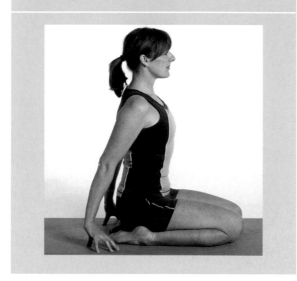

### Aims and usage

To stretch the anterior tibial area on the front of the shin

### Starting position and instructions

Have your client kneel on a gym mat in bare feet. They should keep their heels together and sit back onto them, trying to flatten the tops of their feet to the floor. Have them hold the stretched position for 5–10 seconds and then release.

### Variations

• If your client is unable to flatten their feet completely, place a folded towel between the floor and the front of their ankle. Gradually reduce the thickness of the towel as their flexibility increases.
• To increase the stretch on their toe extensor muscles, place a folded towel beneath the ends of their toes so they are bent (flexed). Again, have them sit back onto their heels.

### Points to note

Your client may allow their ankle to move apart (inversion), which slightly reduces the stretch on the inside of their foot and places a rotation stress (torsion) onto their knee. Have them try to keep their heels together to maintain optimal lower limb alignment.

### Clinical scenario – shin splints

Shin splints may occur in one of three main leg compartments. Pain on the outside (lateral compartment) commonly affects the peroneal muscles while pain close to the inside of the shin bone normally affects the tibialis posterior and big toe flexor muscle. Anterior tibial syndrome is the more common type of shin pain and this affects the tibialis anterior muscle, which pulls the foot upwards and increases arch height. The anterior tibial stretch, kneeling (Exercise 9.9) is useful to reduce pain and tension in the muscle and heel walking (Exercise 9.10) is used to gradually build muscle endurance to enable your client to run for a longer period before pain begins. Foot muscle exercises are also important to build the springy resilience of the foot muscles and exercises such as foot shortening (Exercise 9.1) and toe spread (Exercise 9.2) can begin this process. Walking in bare feet is also helpful to strengthen the foot.

## Exercise 9.10 Heel walking

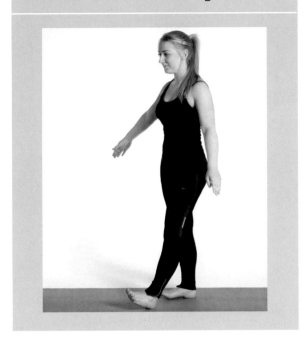

### Aims and usage
To increase muscle endurance of the anterior tibial muscles

### Starting position and instructions
Begin with your client standing in a clear floor space in bare feet. Have them lift their foot from the toes (plantarflex) and walk forwards on their heels. They should take 10 steps and then lower their toes to rest.

### Variations
• To vary the stress imposed on the tissues have your client practise walking backwards and side to side as well.
• Build muscle endurance by increasing the number of steps taken and/or having your client walk more slowly to build up muscle holding time.

### Points to note
Building endurance within the tibialis anterior muscles can be useful in cases of shin splints at the front of the leg (anterior tibial syndrome).

# 10

# // SHOULDER

## ANATOMY REFRESHER

The upper limb consists of several bones. The shoulder blade (*scapula*) is a flat bone lying on the back of the ribcage. At its outer (lateral) end it narrows into a shallow socket (glenoid cavity) which forms a joint with the ball at the top of the upper arm bone (humerus). This joint (glenohumeral joint) is the true shoulder. The scapula is held away from the side of the body by the collar bone (clavicle), which forms a strut. The clavicle itself forms two joints, one with the scapula, the AC or acromioclavicular joint, the other with the breastbone (sternum), the SC or sternoclavicular joint (*see* Figure 10.1).

The AC joint is commonly injured in rugby in a condition called sprung shoulder, while the SC joint may be overstretched and inflamed during exercises such as dips or push-ups in the gym. Most of the bones are superficial and so easily palpated (*see* Figure 10.2).

The superficial nature of the bones makes padding important in exercise therapy. When lying your client on their back on the floor make sure they have a mat or folded towel beneath the whole of their shoulder.

The scapula is not fixed to the ribcage, but held in place by the balanced pull of muscles attaching

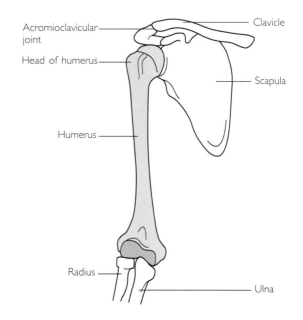

**Figure 10.1** The shoulder joint

to it. On its undersurface lies the *subscapularis* muscle while on the back of the scapula the *supraspinatus* and *infraspinatus* muscles are positioned above and below the scapular spine – a ridge of bone dividing the scapula into two. These small muscles together with the *teres minor* form a group called the *rotator cuff*, which lies beneath the powerful trapezius muscle spanning

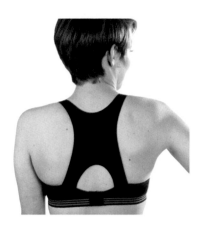

**Figure 10.2** Most of the shoulder bones are superficial.

from the neck out to the shoulders and back into the centre of the spine.

As you move your arm away from your side, both the upper arm bone (humerus) and the shoulder blade (scapula) move in a precise way. This action is known as scapulohumeral rhythm and it is best described in three phases (*see* Table 10.1). Phase one is from the resting position to 30 degrees abduction. At this stage the scapula should remain firmly fixed (stabilised) to the ribcage, forming a firm surface for the arm to move on. As the arms moves out to the side, the large boney knobble at its top (greater tuberosity) can strike the roof of the joint (acromion process). To avoid this, at the beginning of phase 2 abduction (30–90 degrees) the arm rotates outwards (known as 'lateral rotation of the humerus'), allowing the greater tuberosity to pass behind the acromion.

In addition, the acromion moves away from the approaching humerus bone by the scapula twisting outwards and upwards (known as 'lateral scapular rotation'). The two movements are vital to prevent one bone striking the other and trapping tissue between them. When they do meet, a condition called 'shoulder impingement' occurs, which is extremely painful and inflamed (capsulitis) and can lead to the joint becoming stiff and eventually seizing up completely as a frozen shoulder. During phase 3 of shoulder abduction (from 90 degrees to full range overhead) the humerus continues to move outwards while the scapula is drawn round and to the side of the trunk. This action requires the upper spine (thoracic region) to flatten, a situation which sometimes may not occur if it is very stiff. Where thoracic stiffness is present, the arm cannot be lifted overhead without it coming forwards as well.

| Table 10.1 | Scapulohumeral rhythm | |
|---|---|---|
| **Phase 1**<br>*Rest to 30°*<br>*abduction* | **Phase 2**<br>*30–90°*<br>*abduction* | **Phase 3**<br>*90° to*<br>*full range* |
| • Scapula fixed to ribcage | • Humeral laterally rotates<br>• Scapula twist up and out | • Humerus abducts<br>• Scapula drawn to side of trunk<br>• Thoracic spine flattens |

## Exercise 10.1 Scapular stability – passive repositioning

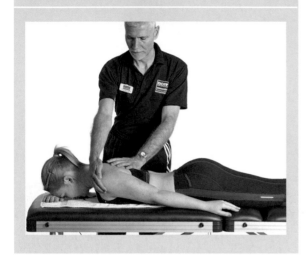

### Aims and usage
To re-educate the scapular stabilising muscles

### Starting position and instructions
Begin with your client lying on their front. Place one cupped hand over the front/outer (anterolateral) aspect of the shoulder, the other flat hand over the scapula. Gently draw the scapula back and downwards (retraction and depression). Ask your client to hold the position for 3–5 seconds and then relax. Repeat the action, asking your client to follow the movement with their scapula (active movement). Gradually apply less force to move the scapula so that your client contributes more to the action.

### Variations
• Apply greater force in cases where the scapula is drawn forwards by tight anterior structures rather than allow to move forwards by lax scapular stabilisers.

• Where the shoulder elevators (upper trapezius) are tight, apply greater force drawing the scapula downwards (known as 'depression') rather than backwards.

### Points to note
The scapula is held onto the ribcage by a balance of pull from the serratus anterior and trapezius muscles (lower fibres especially). Laxity in these muscles allows the scapula to drop forwards in the lying position or downwards in the standing position.

## Exercise 10.2 Scapular stability – active repositioning

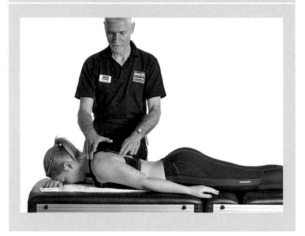

### Aims and usage
To re-educate active control of the scapular stabilising muscles

### Starting position and instructions
Begin with your client lying on their front. Place one cupped hand over the anterolateral aspect of the shoulder, the other flat hand over the scapula. Initially perform a passive action by gently drawing

the scapula back and downwards (retraction and depression). Repeat the action, asking your client to follow the movement with their scapula (active movement), gradually applying less passive force so your client takes over the movement. Release your hands and place one finger close to the bottom/inner aspect (inferior angle) of their scapula and encourage them to press their scapula against this point (tactile cueing).

## Variations

• Once your client is familiar with the action you may dispense with the passive action and focus on them moving their scapula down and in towards your guiding finger placed at the inferior angle of the scapula.

• Your client may self-monitor this action for home exercise. Ask them to place their opposite hand behind their back and place their thumb in the position of your fingers. They then press the inferior angle of their scapula against their own thumb. Where they do not have the flexibility to reach behind their back, they should ask their partner to monitor the action with their fingers.

## Points to note

• Have your client perform scapular stability – passive repositioning (Exercise 10.1) before using this exercise. Have them perform the exercise in a variety of starting positions including lying, sitting and standing.

---

### Exercise 10.3 Cat paws

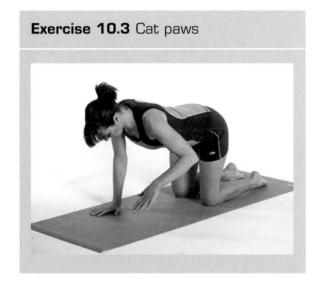

### Aims and usage

To maintain scapular stability and alignment during arm movement

### Starting position and instructions

Begin with your client kneeling with their shoulders directly over their hands and hips directly over their knees (in box position). Ensure they focus on their shoulder alignment, opening their chest and drawing their scapulae gently downwards and inwards so they lie flat on their ribcage. Have them maintain this position as they lift one hand up from the floor, bending their elbow but maintaining the position of their trunk. Have them hold the position for 1–2 seconds and then replace their hand and perform the same action with their opposite shoulder, performing 8–10 reps on each shoulder alternately.

### Variations

• When your client has lifted their hand from the floor, ensure they maintain scapular alignment while moving their arm forward and backwards or side to side by 10–15cm only.

129

• If your client tends to dip their shoulder down as they lift their hand from the floor, place a book or yoga block across their shoulders and ask them to aim to keep this horizontal throughout the exercise (tactile cueing).

## Points to note
Your client's attention should be focused on the position of their scapula rather than the movement of their arm.

---

### Exercise 10.4 Knee press-ups

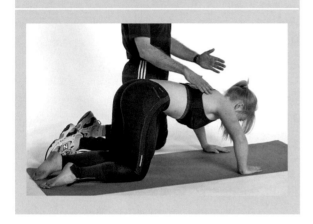

## Aims and usage
To maintain scapular stability and alignment during weight-bearing arm movement

## Starting position and instructions
Begin with your client kneeling on all fours (in box position) with their shoulders over their hands and their hips over their knees. Have them open their chest to flatten their thoracic spine. They should then bend their elbows by 20–30 degrees, keeping their chest open and avoiding rounding their upper back (thoracic flexion).

## Variations
• Have your client move their body forwards so their hip flexion angle is increased (hips forward of knees). Holding this leg position, have them bend their knees as before.
• Instead of bending their elbows, have them keep them locked and sway their body from side to side, keeping their scapulae firmly on their ribcage, avoiding any swinging.

## Points to note
The aim of this exercise is to maintain scapular stability so that the scapulae remain flat against the ribcage throughout the movement. If the inner (medial) edge, or lower (inferior) angle of the scapula lifts, stop the exercise and have your client reposition their scapula flat against the ribcage before repeating the exercise using less arm movement.

## Exercise 10.5 Sitting sternal lift

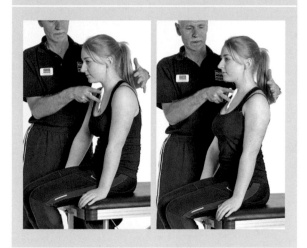

### Aims and usage

To encourage thoracic spine extension in sitting while maintaining scapular alignment

### Starting position and instructions

Have your client sit on a firm chair or gym bench with their feet flat on the floor. Ask them to lift their breastbone (sternum) and at the same time draw their shoulder blades downwards. They should hold the position for 10–15 seconds (isometric hold) and then repeat.

### Variations

• Have your client perform the exercise with their back against a wall to avoid body sway and give feedback (tactile feedback) about shoulder position.
• Have them place their hands onto the bench at their sides (if they do not reach the bench use two blocks/books beneath them). Ask them to gently press their hands down (shoulder depression) as they lift their sternum.

### Points to note

The aim of this movement is to perform thoracic spine extension rather than ribcage expansion. Make sure that your client does not simply take a deep breath as they try to lift as this also activates the upper trapezius (shoulder elevation or shrug) when the lower trapezius (shoulder depression) is the muscle we are aiming to work.

### Clinical scenario – recovery from shoulder surgery

Various types of shoulder surgery may be performed with one of the most common being treatment for trapped tissue (shoulder impingement), which gives sudden 'tweaks' of pain as the arm is lifted towards the horizontal. Following surgery, movement and strength need to be regained gradually, taking care not to disrupt the healing tissues. The hospital physiotherapist will advise initial exercise and after these have been completed home rehab can be progressed. Initially, scapular stability and alignment is emphasised using scapular stability – passive (Exercise 10.1) and then active repositioning (Exercise 10.2). Once alignment is good use cat paws (Exercise 10.3) to place alternating load on the shoulder while maintaining the aligned position. Strength is progressed using the knee press-up (Exercise 10.4) and further using the seated row (Exercise 10.15), emphasising downward (depression) and backward (retraction) motion of the shoulder blade. Arm actions are begun using simple forward and side motions which are then performed resisted using pulley triplanar arm abduction (Exercise 10.13).

## Exercise 10.6 Overhead reach lying

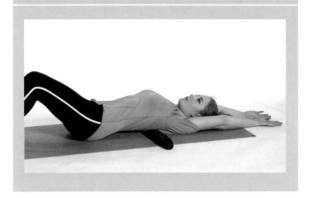

### Aims and usage

To stretch the thoracic spine into extension and expand the ribcage

### Starting position and instructions

Begin by placing a rolled towel beneath your client's shoulder blades, facing across the body. Have them bend their knees to flatten their lower back and lie back onto the towel. Ask them to reach overhead with their straight arms using the leverage of their arms to press their upper spine onto the towel. They should hold the fully stretched position for 20–30 seconds and then release.

### Variations

• Use a thin (10cm) foam roller or half roll instead of a rolled towel.
• Instead of your client applying overpressure using their arms, have them keep their arms at their sides and lie on the towel for 5–10 minutes. This action uses the bodyweight to slowly stretch the tissues of the back.

### Points to note

Stiffness of the upper back can come from soft tissue tightness, bone position and bone shape. This action stretches soft tissues and helps to realign the thoracic spine, reducing the curvature (or kyphosis). It does not affect bone shape. In cases of osteoporosis, the action may still be useful to target the soft tissue adaptation that occurs in parallel to bone changes. Less overpressure is required, however, and initially it may be necessary to support the body in a flexed position with cushions. As flexibility increases, less cushions are required.

## Exercise 10.7 Wall walking

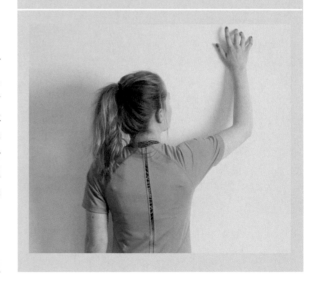

### Aims and usage

To increase range of motion at the shoulder without taking full arm weight

### Starting position and instructions

Begin with your client standing facing a wall. Have them place their hand on the wall at shoulder level and walk their fingers up the wall, stopping if they begin to shrug their shoulder (scapular elevation).

## Variations

• Have your client stand side-on to the wall to work pure abduction, and partial side-on for flexion-abduction.

• Have them place their other hand over their shoulder close to their neck (upper trapezius) to monitor and prevent shoulder shrugging.

## Points to note

The aim of this action is to work abduction of the shoulder (glenohumeral) joint. In cases of frozen shoulder, glenohumeral movement decreases and, to compensate, movement of the shoulder blade (scapular thoracic movement) increases. Try to reduce scapular thoracic movement by having your client avoid shoulder shrugging. They should aim to take as much arm weight as possible through their fingers on the wall to encourage free movement of the joint with less muscle guarding.

### Exercise 10.8 Mobilisation with movement

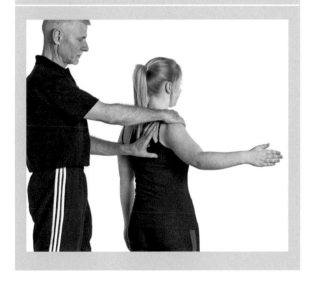

## Aims and usage

To encourage correct alignment of the shoulder region during an arm abduction movement

## Starting position and instructions

Begin with your client standing with you behind them. Place your cupped hand over their shoulder and draw the ball of the shoulder gently back. Then have your client lift their arm out sideways (abduction) and point their thumb upwards (outward rotation). At the same time you draw their shoulder back, preventing it from moving forwards into a round shouldered position.

## Variations

• To create greater force, use a belt placed around the front of your client's shoulder. They should loop the belt around themselves, and lean back slightly to create force with their bodyweight rather than their hands.

• Have your client perform the exercise close to a wall, to take some of their arm weight through the wall by sweeping their arm across the wall surface.

## Points to note

You should guide the position of your client's shoulder rather than force it. If they have pain in their shoulder when they move, the action of drawing the shoulder back should ease the pain.

## 10.9 Side lying arm abduction

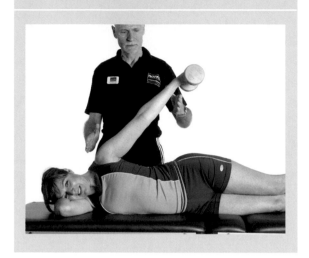

### Aims and usage
To work the shoulder abductor muscles with reducing leverage

### Starting position and instructions
Begin with your client lying on their side with a small (1–2kg) dumbbell in their hand. Have them keep their arm straight and begin with their arm at their side. They should then lift their arm from the horizontal position (at their side) to the vertical position (pointing to the ceiling) and then lower.

### Variations
• Have your client bend their elbow to reduce stress on the elbow joint in cases of elbow injury.
• To reduce resistance and leverage, do not have them use a dumbbell, but instead get them to place their hand over their shoulder and lift their arm leading with their elbow (short lever resistance).

### Points to note
This exercise makes use of the fact that leverage is greatest in a horizontal position. In standing because the arm is vertical when by your side, leverage increases as you lift your arm upwards to the horizontal. In this case the resistance is *increasing* as your shoulder muscles are shortening. In the side-lying position used in this exercise the situation is reversed. Now, the position of maximum leverage is at the start of the exercise (arm by your side) as the arm is horizontal. As you lift, your arm approaches the vertical position so leverage is *reducing*. Now the resistance is reducing as your shoulder muscles shorten.

### Exercise 10.10 Side lying lateral arm rotation

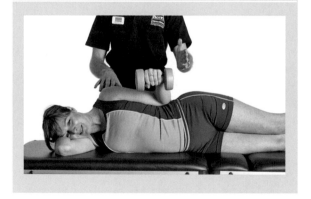

### Aims and usage
To work the shoulder lateral rotator muscles in isolation from the larger chest and shoulder muscles

### Starting position and instructions
Begin with your client lying on their side with a small (1–2kg) dumbbell gripped in their hand. Have them bend their elbow to 90 degrees and

pull their upper arm close into their side, allowing their forearm to rest close to the vertical near their abdomen. Ensuring they keep their upper arm pressed to their side, ask them to twist their arm bone (humeral rotation) so that their forearm moves in an arc to end up near vertical pointing to the ceiling. They should hold the position for 1–2 seconds before lowering under control.

## Variations
To work the inner range position only, have your client begin with their forearm resting horizontally in front of their chest on a gym bench or small stack of yoga blocks.

## Points to note
In many cases of shoulder pain, the range of lateral rotation is limited because the medial rotator muscles are very tight. This exercise can then be used as a useful stretching exercise (dynamic stretch) by choosing a light weight and pressing the arm further into range at the end of the movement as the arm points towards the ceiling.

---

**Exercise 10.11** Sitting shoulder press with stick

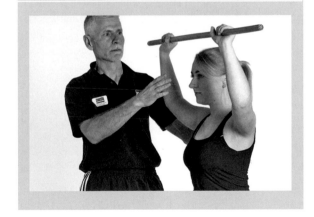

### Aims and usage
To increase combined range of both abduction and lateral rotation movements

### Starting position and instructions
Begin with your client holding a stick (broom handle) in their hands about 1m apart. Have them hold the centre of the stick on or close to their breastbone (sternum). They should drop their elbows down towards their sides. From this starting position, they then press the stick upwards, trying to keep it in close to their body so that it passes close to their face. Encourage them to try to fully lock their elbows out at the top of the movement and then lower back to their breastbone again.

### Variations
• To increase the range of lateral rotation place the bar across their shoulders and have them press and lower from this point rather than their breastbone. When using a barbell, this variation is called press behind neck and is a separate exercise to the sitting shoulder press described above.
• Have them place their hands closer together, to just brush their shoulders. The action now is a more vertical press directly upwards compared to the original position with hands 1m apart, where the action is upwards and slightly outwards.

### Points to note
This exercise requires adequate shoulder flexibility to be able to keep the bar close into the body. Where shoulder flexibility is limited

there is a tendency to allow the bar to move forwards so that the press action is in an arc rather than a vertical line. If this occurs, your client should keep using a very light resistance (thin wooden stick) until they are able to perform the vertical action. Once this is mastered, more resistance can be used (metal weight bar) to build up strength.

### Exercise 10.12 Shoulder press standing

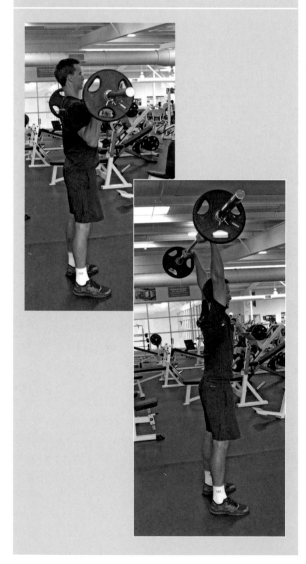

### Aims and usage
To build shoulder strength and power using a functional overhead press action

### Starting position and instructions
Begin with your client holding a barbell undergrasp (palms up) gripping the bar just wider than their shoulders. Ask them to rest the bar on the top of their breastbone. They should then press the bar upwards in a straight line so that it passes close to their face. As the bar passes overhead, they should press their head forwards slightly so that the bar path continues in a vertical line. Have them lower the bar under control back to its resting position.

### Variations
• To create momentum in the bar have your client dip their legs (bend knees and hips) slightly at the beginning of the action. As the bar begins to move, keep the movement going upwards by having them press with their arms. They should not dip their legs to move the bar up and then allow it to fall before they press with their arms.
• Have your client place the bar across their shoulders and press the bar from this position (press behind neck exercise). As the bar is behind the head, this action avoids excessive spinal extension.

### Points to note
In this exercise the bar path must be vertical. If the bar moves forwards or backwards, it will become unsteady and may pull your client off balance.

## Exercise 10.13 Pulley triplanar arm abduction

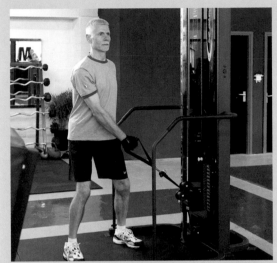

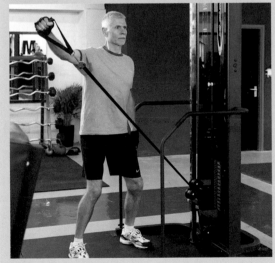

### Aims and usage

To work the shoulder musculature in triplane motion

### Starting position and instructions

Begin with your client standing side-on to a low pulley machine. They should then grasp the 'D' handle of the machine and pull the handle upwards (flexion) and outwards to the side (abduction) while twisting their arm from the starting position where the knuckles face upwards to the finish where the knuckles face backwards (lateral rotation).

### Variations

• Use a high pulley and have your client stand facing and slightly to the side of the machine. Have them pull the handle down (extension) towards themselves (adduction) and move their hand from the knuckles back position to the knuckles up position (medial rotation).

• Have them stand with their back to the machine and take one step forwards so their arm is held back. They should lift the handle forwards (flexion), outwards (abduction) and turn their hand from a knuckles up position to a knuckles out position (lateral rotation).

### Points to note

Triplanar motions are movements that occur in all three movement planes – sagittal, frontal and transverse. They are more functional in that they mimic what the body does in day-to-day activities. Many modern weight training machines restrict users to unilateral (e.g. flexion-extension) or bilateral (e.g. flexion-abduction) motions. These types of simpler actions are useful at the start of rehabilitation because they are easier to control. It is important to progress to more functional actions towards the end of rehab to prepare a user to return to normal activities at work or within sport.

## Clinical scenario – frozen shoulder

Frozen shoulder is a condition in which the capsule of the joint tightens and leaves the shoulder tight and painful. The condition progresses through various stages dictated by pain and limitation of movement, but can last for up to two years in many cases. Depending on severity, treatment ranges from physiotherapy to surgical capsular release. Exercise is particularly important in the stages when pain begins to ease. Both the amount and quality of movement at the shoulder needs to be improved. Overhead reach lying (Exercise 10.6) is useful as it uses the weight and leverage of the arms to encourage further movement in a relatively protected position. As movement eases, wall walking (Exercise 10.7) is helpful to encourage functional use of the newly gained motion. The focus must be on movement quality as well as range because in frozen shoulder clients tend to compensate for stiffness at the shoulder joint (glenohumeral joint) by moving excessively at the shoulder blade (scapular-thoracic joint). Encourage good alignment and avoidance of shoulder shrugging as the arm is lifted. 'Mobilisation with movement' is a technique which combines movement with guidance from the therapist or training partner and is especially useful in this condition.

Re-strengthening has to be in a position which does not cause pain. Side lying arm abduction (Exercise 10.9) is helpful here as the leverage of the arm reduces as the arm is lifted, effectively lowering the resistance as the arm is lifted towards a potentially painful angle. Side lying lateral arm rotation (Exercise 10.10) is an important exercise in many shoulder conditions as it targets the rotator cuff muscles, which are important to shoulder movement quality. If these muscles are weaker, the quality of movement at the shoulder suffers. When movement and strength begin to return, actions such as sitting shoulder press with stick (Exercise 10.11) are helpful to form a bridge between pure rehab exercise and return to the gym.

## Exercise 10.14 Press-up walking flat

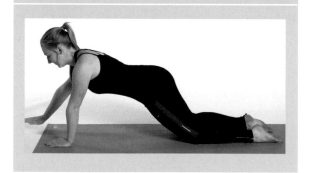

### Aims and usage

To introduce intermittent loading on the shoulder joint

### Starting position and instructions

Begin with your client in the press-up position, either with legs straight (full press-up) or knees on the floor (partial press-up). Have them place their hands directly beneath their shoulders and open their chest by extending the thoracic spine and drawing their shoulder blades back and down slightly so they are flat against the ribcage, to focus on scapular stability. As they maintain optimal shoulder alignment, ask them to walk their hands forwards and backwards by about 10–15cm with each 'step'.

### Variations

•   Instead of walking their hands forwards and

backwards (flexion-extension), have them move them from side to side (abduction-adduction).
• Have them lie facing a step or low gym bench and walk the hands onto and off this with each step.
• Use a mobile platform such as a balance board, BOSU® or vibrating platform to step the hands onto. This challenges shoulder proprioception.

## Points to note
The hip is a ball and socket joint built for stability rather than a large range of motion and designed to take weight (compression load)

during standing, walking and running. The shoulder is also a ball and socket, but built more for mobility than stability. This design difference leads many therapists to focus on movement range and strength of the shoulder but to forget joint loading. This is a mistake, because pressing actions in day-to-day activities and falls onto the hand in sports such as rugby involve substantial joint loading at the shoulder. This type of exercise is useful towards the end of a rehabilitation programme to prepare a client for return to work and/or sport.

## Exercise 10.15 Seated row

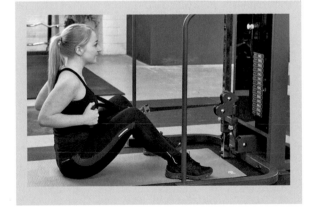

## Aims and usage
To work the shoulder retractor muscles

## Starting position and instructions
Begin with your client sitting in front of a low pulley or specialised seated row machine. Have them bend their knees slightly to release tension in their hamstring muscles and enable their pelvis to tilt forwards (anterior tilt) so they can sit upright without rounding their lumbar spine.

They should then grasp the bar shoulder-width apart and pull it in towards the centre of their breastbone (sternum). Have them pause in this position and then release the bar under control.

## Variations
• Rather than a straight bar, you may use a specialised rowing handle (double 'D' handle). With a straight bar your client's knuckles face upwards (forearms pronated) but with a rowing handle their knuckles face to the side (forearms midway between pronation and supination).
• Have them take the bar to their waist or chin to vary the muscle work.

## Points to note
This action should be a combination of scapular retraction (moving the shoulder blades together) and scapular depression (moving the shoulder blades downwards). There is sometimes a tendency to shrug the shoulders (scapular elevation) which should be avoided, as it emphasises the upper portion of the trapezius muscle when the mid and lower portions are the target for this exercise.

# ELBOW, WRIST AND HAND

# 11

## ANATOMY REFRESHER

The elbow consist of three joints. The upper arm bone (humerus) forms joints with both the bone on the thumb side of the forearm (radius) and the bone on the little finger side of the forearm (ulna). The two forearm bones also form a joint to allow the radius bone to twist. Your elbow can therefore bend and straighten (flexion and extension) and swivel to face your palm down (pronation) or up (supination). Often following injury there is a focus on getting back the bending and straightening actions of the elbow with little regard to pronation and supination. These are vital movements because without them the position of the wrist and hand change considerably, often leading to poor grip.

The forearm muscles are all long and lean and their tendons come together to attach to knobbles of bone on the inside and outside of the elbow. The inside of the forearm is called the common flexor origin (CFO) and the outside the common extensor origin (CEO), and both are involved in injuries to the elbow. The size of the grip affects tension in the forearm muscles, a consideration when using weight training, for example. Gripping a narrower object such as a weight training bar causes the forearm extensors on the back of the forearm to be wound more tightly, increasing stress on the CFO, a common cause of tennis elbow (known as 'extensor tendinopathy'). To reduce stress on the tissues while using the same weight, make the bar fatter by having your client wear a padded weight training glove or wrapping a layer of foam rubber around the bar.

The wrist consists of joints between the ends of the forearm bones (radius and ulna) and the block-like hand (carpal) bones, and between the individual carpal bones themselves. Each joint is strengthened by ligaments and controlled by muscles travelling from the forearm to the fingers. On the underside (palmar aspect), the carpal bones form a shallow curve that is covered by a fibrous band (flexor retinaculum). Together this structure is called the carpal tunnel, and through it run the long finger bending tendons (flexors) and the median nerve. Compression of the nerve within the tunnel causes carpal tunnel syndrome, described below (*see* Figure 11.1).

Movement of the wrist joint following injury can often be severely limited by hardened swelling (known as 'consolidated oedema'), tight tissue and bone changes where a break (fracture) has occurred. Exercise is important to restore some or all movement and even in cases where the whole movement range cannot be regained, restoring just a small portion can significantly reduce pain and improve function.

The main function of the fingers is to grip, and two categories of grip occur. Precision grip is applied using the tips, pads and nails of the fingers working together as pincers. Power grip involves the whole hand. The wrist muscles work together to lock the wrist and the fingers and thumb work together to pull the object into the centre of the palm.

A balance should exist between the finger bending muscles (flexors) and finger straightening muscles (extensors) so that the wrist stays straight as you grip. Often the extensor muscles are weaker than the flexors, causing the wrist to angle inwards, leaving you at risk of overuse conditions of the forearm and elbow.

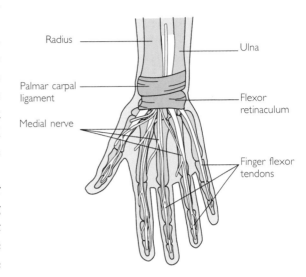

**Figure 11.1** The wrist joint

## Exercise 11.1 Resisted wrist extension

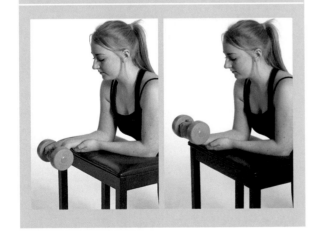

### Aims and usage
To build strength and endurance in the wrist extensor muscles

### Starting position and instructions
Begin with your client's forearm supported on a high bench or table, with their hand over the table edge. Have them hold a small (2kg) dumbbell in their hand, knuckled up. Ask them to allow their wrist to flex, taking the weight towards the floor, and then extend their wrist, taking the weight towards the ceiling.

### Variations
• Have your client perform the exercise using a resistance band or tubing instead of a dumbbell.
• Rather than them resting their forearm on a table, have them support it using their other hand cupped on the lower forearm close to their wrist.

### Points to note
In cases of tendinopathy (tennis elbow), the aim

of rehabilitation is to stimulate the healing tissue to adapt to the higher stresses imposed though exercise. The emphasis is on higher resistance with eccentric actions (wrist lowering to flexion) being important. Tendinopathy can affect both the muscle going above the elbow (extensor carpi radialis longus) and the one ending just below (extensor carpi radialis brevis). Where pain occurs above the elbow the exercise is better practised with the elbow straight to target the higher muscle.

## Exercise 11.2 Arm curl

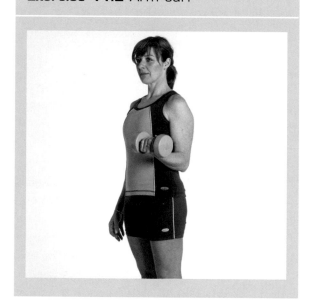

### Aims and usage

To strengthen the arm flexor muscles

### Starting position and instructions

Begin with your client standing with a dumbbell or other weight (e.g. food can) held in their hand, knuckles down. Keeping their arm tucked into their side, have them bend their elbow until their hand comes close to their shoulder before lowering their arm again until it is straight.

### Variations

• Have your client begin with their knuckles facing up, and as they bend their arm they should twist (supinate) their forearm to turn their knuckles down.
• Have them rest their upper arm on an angled bench to prevent it moving as they bend their arm (preacher curl exercise).
• Have them perform the exercise using a barbell held in both hands. They should curl (bend) the elbow until the bar touches the top of their breast-bone and then lower back to the top of their thighs.

### Points to note

The arm curl action (elbow flexion) is carried out in the main by the brachialis, brachioradialis and biceps muscles. As well as bending the arm, the biceps also supinates the forearm, an action countered by the pronator teres muscle in daily actions. To emphasise the biceps in the arm curl exercise, we work elbow flexion and supination, while to emphasise the brachioradialis, we perform the curl with the forearm in mid-position (thumb upwards).

The biceps muscle also flexes the shoulder, so full work of the muscle as part of the rehabilitation following biceps rupture, for example, involves a combined action of shoulder and elbow flexion with forearm supination, drawing the hand towards the mouth (known as 'humeral internal rotation'). This sequence of movements is called a *feeding pattern*.

## Exercise 11.3 Triceps extension overhead

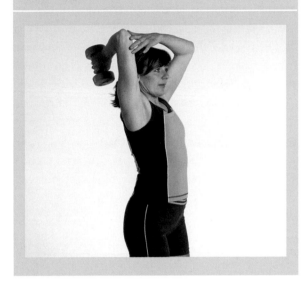

### Aims and usage
To strengthen the triceps muscles using an overhead action

### Starting position and instructions
Begin with your client standing with a small dumbbell or weight (e.g. food can) held in their right hand. They should then reach overhead and bend their elbow so their hand rests level with the base of their neck. They can support their upper arm using their cupped left hand. Then ask them to straighten their right arm without allowing their elbow to move forwards. Have them pause in the straight arm (elbow locked) position and then lower their hand again until it rests on their shoulder.

### Variations
Have your client perform the exercise with both hands, holding the dumbbell handle between the thumb webs of both hands so that the two together form an 'O'. Ensure they keep their elbows close to the sides of their head (shoulder adduction) as they straighten their arms – do not allow them to let their elbows splay apart (shoulder abduction).

### Points to note
The triceps muscle works over the elbow and the shoulder to extend both joints. This exercise mimics the muscle action of an overhead throw in sport, or overhead reach in daily living, for example, reaching to the top shelf of a high cupboard.

## Exercise 11.4 Triceps kickback

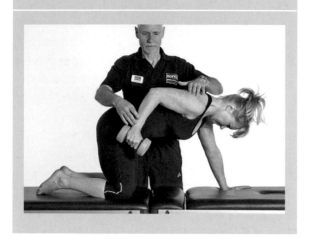

### Aims and usage

To work the triceps muscle with maximum leverage at full inner range

### Starting position and instructions

Begin with your client kneeling on a gym bench with one leg straight on the floor. Have them hold a dumbbell in their right hand and tuck their upper arm into the side of their body. They should then extend their elbow, keeping their upper arm horizontal until they lock their elbow out straight. Have them hold this position for 1–2 seconds and then lower the weight, bending their elbow back to the 90 degree starting position.

### Variations

Have your client perform the exercise using resistance tubing or a band, with the band held in the hand and the other end attached to the front leg of the bench on the same side.

### Points to note

This action in some ways is the opposite of triceps extension overhead (Exercise 11.3). In the triceps kickback, the triceps is at its shortest position when the elbow is locked and the arm is horizontal (maximum leverage). In the triceps extension overhead, the muscle is shortest when the arm is vertical (minimum leverage). Shortening the muscle with maximum overload in this way is using a bodybuilding technique called 'peak contraction', where a muscle is squeezed tightly at the end-range of increased overload.

## Exercise 11.5 Triceps extension on pulley

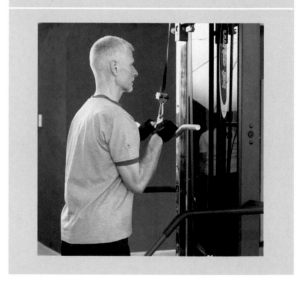

### Aims and usage

To strengthen the arm extensor muscles (triceps and anconeus) using elbow movement alone

## Starting position and instructions

Begin with your client facing a high pulley machine. Have them grip (knuckles up) the bar of the machine, placing one hand each side of the cable attachment to the handle. They should tuck their elbows into the side of their body and, keeping their upper arms still, press the bar downwards, straightening their arms as they do so to lift the weight up from the weight stack. Have them pause in the lower position and then slowly bend their arms again to lower the weight back onto the stack.

## Variations

• Have your client perform the action single handed using a 'D' handle attached to the high pulley. As they press with their right hand, they should support their right upper arm in their cupped left hand to fix the upper arm and prevent unwanted movement.

• Have them use an angled bar or rope attached to a high pulley to alter their grip angle. With a straight bar the forearm is held pronated throughout the exercise, but with an angled bar or rope attachment the forearm is positioned midway between pronation and supination, which some users find more comfortable.

## Points to note

When one arm is considerably weaker than the other, using a single handed action can be useful because the different resistances on each arm help to regain equal strength.

### Clinical scenario – tennis elbow

Tennis elbow (lateral epicondylitis) is a condition affecting the attachment of the forearm extensor muscles (pulling the wrist upwards) to the lower end of the humerus bone just above the elbow joint. It occurs through overuse and especially when gripping objects with the wrist locked. The muscle attachment known as the common extensor origin is a pencil-thin band that thickens and toughens, changing its blood flow in cases of tennis elbow. The result is pain when objects are gripped at an awkward angle. Various treatments are available, and exercise therapy is important to build up the endurance of the forearm extensor muscles. Use resisted wrist extension (Exercise 11.1) to build endurance, using a light resistance (weight or band) while having your client perform high numbers of reps (20–25) and also using lower reps but increasing the duration of each rep (10–20 seconds). Resisted pronation/supination (Exercise 11.8) can also help, especially in those whose jobs involve using screwdrivers and spanners. Power grip using ball (Exercise 11.11) is useful to build grip endurance. Have your client grip to the onset of elbow pain and then release and allow the pain to subside completely before repeating. The aim is to increase the time your client can hold the grip before pain begins.

## Exercise 11.6 Bench dip

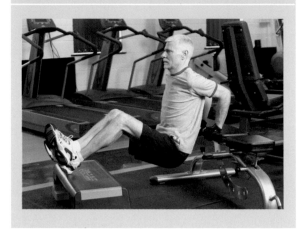

### Aims and usage
To work the elbow and shoulder extensor muscles in a joint loaded format

### Starting position and instructions
Have your client place a gym bench against a wall to prevent it from slipping and begin with the heels of their hands gripping the edge of the bench, hands close together. Have them place their heels on the floor, hip-width apart, with their legs out straight. Keeping their elbows close, ask them to bend their arms to lower their buttocks vertically towards the floor and then press back upwards again.

### Variations
• To increase the workload and have your client take a greater amount of their bodyweight through their arms, have them place their heels up on a bench rather than on the floor.
• To increase the workload by adding external resistance, have them place a weight plate (disc) on their lap.

• To reduce the workload, have them take less of their bodyweight through their arms by bending their knees to 90 degrees.

### Points to note
• The action should be to lower the buttocks directly downwards so that they brush the edge of the bench. Do not allow the buttocks to move forwards.
• To focus work onto the triceps make sure your client keeps their elbows close together rather than allowing them to splay apart. Where the elbows move apart, extra work is placed onto the shoulder adductor muscles to hold the arms in position.

## Exercise 11.7 Chin-up

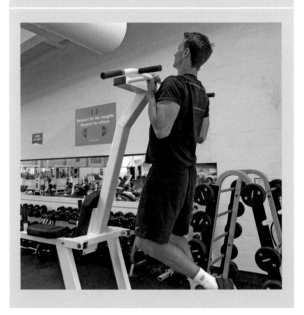

### Aims and usage
To work the arm and shoulder muscles in a functional overhead pulling action

## Starting position and instructions

Begin with your client standing in front of a high bar. Have them hold the bar (knuckles upwards) keeping their arms shoulder-width apart. They should pull their body towards the bar until their chin touches or passes over the bar, and then lower under control.

## Variations

• Have your client bend their knees and while you or their training partner partially lifts them upwards, they lower their body under their own control, which emphasises the eccentric portion of the exercise.

• Instead of a high bar, use a high pulley with a straight bar attached. Gradually progress the exercise using more blocks on the weight stack until your client is able to select a weight that almost causes them to lift from the floor. At this point they should be strong enough to transfer to the high bar chin described above.

• Have them perform the exercise with a wide grip to increase emphasis on the shoulder adductor muscles.

## Points to note

Lifting the whole bodyweight with your arms is an intense exercise. It is a functional action and one used in sports such as gymnastics, for example, and is often part of a fitness test for Forces personnel. Typically this action is used in bodybuilding workouts and high intensity training (HIT) where few repetitions are performed, but to high intensity. Arm strength has to be proportional to bodyweight, so if your client is overweight, they may find the action too hard.

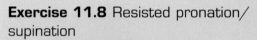

**Exercise 11.8** Resisted pronation/supination

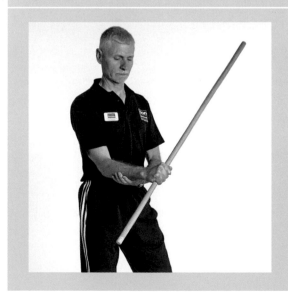

## Aims and usage

To re-strengthen the forearm pronator and supinator muscles following wrist or elbow injury

## Starting position and instructions

Begin with your client standing with their right elbow bent to 90 degrees, arm tucked into the side of their body. Have them hold a lever in their right hand, knuckles down. This may be a hammer, dumbbell with one end weight removed, or simply a stick. They then twist their arm so that the stick moves in a semicircle, moving from a knuckles-down position to a knuckles-up position and then back.

## Variations

Increasing the leverage increases the overload applied during the exercise. Begin with your client holding the stick in the centre for minimum leverage and gradually they move their hands further to one end to increase leverage, causing their forearm muscles to work harder.

## Points to note
The action should be pure forearm pronation and supination without any shoulder movement, which would pull the elbow away from the side of your client's body.

### Exercise 11.9 Flexion/extension closed chain stretch on table

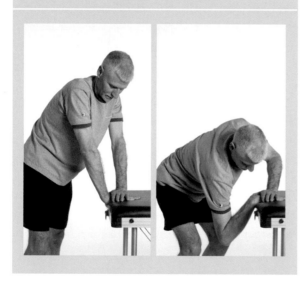

### Aims and usage
To restore mobility to the wrist following injury and swelling (oedema)

### Starting position and instructions
Begin with your client facing a table edge and have them place their right hand flat on the table surface with their wrist crease at the edge. They should place their left hand flat on top of their right with the web space level with the wrist, border of the first finger at the wrist crease. Have them press down with their left hand to

fix their right to the tabletop. Encourage flexion and extension at their right wrist by having them lift and lower their right elbow above and then below the level of the tabletop. When they get to the end of the available movement range in each direction, have them place gentle overpressure on the movement to squeeze slightly further into the stiff movement range.

### Variations
• Where wrist extension is more limited, have your client stand up and press their bodyweight forward over the tabletop.
• Where wrist flexion is limited, have them squat or kneel down and pull their elbow down beneath the table.

### Points to note
This action uses the leverage of the forearm and the bodyweight to force extra movement at the wrist. It is useful where a client has thick, settled swelling (known as 'consolidated oedema'), but must be used progressively, first applying gentle pressure and then increasing each day as the wrist allows. If your client's wrist is very sore afterwards, have them practise every other day and use less force during the movement.

EXERCISE THERAPY

## Exercise 11.10 Abduction/adduction closed chain stretch on table

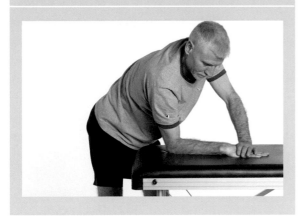

### Aims and usage

To restore mobility to the wrist following injury and swelling (oedema)

### Starting position and instructions

Begin with your client facing a table edge and have them place their right hand flat on the table surface with the wrist crease at the edge. They should place their left hand flat on top of their right with the web space level with the wrist, border of the first finger at the wrist crease. Have them press down with their left hand to fix their right to the tabletop. Encourage sideways movement (abduction and adduction) of the wrist, remembering that movement towards the little finger side (ulnar deviation) is less than that towards the thumb side (radial deviation). When your client gets to the end of the available movement range in each direction, have them place gentle overpressure on the movement to squeeze slightly further into the stiff movement range.

### Variations

To increase movement range you can use a number of small presses at the end of the range (pulsing) or a single pressure held for 10–20 seconds (static stretch). Alternate between the two methods to see which works best for your client.

### Points to note

• This action uses the leverage of the forearm and the bodyweight to force extra movement at the wrist. It is useful where your client has thick, settled swelling (known as 'consolidated oedema'), but must be used progressively, first applying gentle pressure and then increasing each day as your client's wrist allows. If their wrist is very sore afterwards, have them practise every other day and use less force during the movement.

• Following wrist fracture the bones may be misshapen so will not move further. Some of the stiffness with the injury will be from thick swelling, some from bone changes. Thick swelling feels rubbery when you press into the limited movement, but bone on bone contact feels hard.

## Exercise 11.11 Power grip using ball

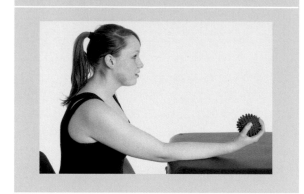

### Aims and usage
To re-strengthen grip following hand injury

### Starting position and instructions
Begin with your client sitting in front of a table with three or four balls of different sizes and consistency, for example, a squash ball, a child's rubber cricket ball, a spiky massage ball or a tennis ball. Have them place the ball in the centre of their palm and grip it, ensuring that all their fingers wrap around the ball and the thumb grips towards the fingers (thumb opposition). They should hold the ball tightly for 5–10 seconds and then release. Ask them to repeat the movement with each different ball.

### Variations
•  Have your client position the ball closer to the thumb and grip using the thumb side (radial) section of the hand in cases where the thumb or index finger has been injured.
•  Have them position the ball closer to the little finger and grip using the little finger side (ulnar) section of the hand where the little (fifth) or index (fourth) fingers have been injured.

### Points to note
Following injury where the knuckle (metacarpophalangeal joint or MCP) or finger (interphalangeal joint or IP) joints have been damaged, it is often difficult to bend the finger around the ball tightly. In this case have your client use their other hand to press the fingers tightly onto the ball and then release and try to maintain grip with the injured hand muscles.

## Exercise 11.12 Precision grip using small objects

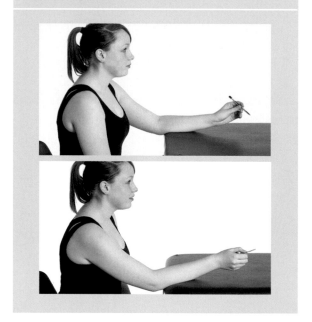

### Aims and usage
To regain strength and precision of the finger muscles following injury

### Starting position and instructions
Begin with your client sitting in front of a table with a number of small objects of different sizes

and consistencies in front of them. Have them grip each object, first between their thumb and index finger, using the tip of each, and then thumb and middle, ring and little fingers. Have them hold each grip for 3–5 seconds and then release.

## Variations

• Have your client grip between the sides of their fingers (scissor grip) rather than the tips.
• Once the object is being gripped, have them use their other hand to try to pull the object out while they grip more strongly (isometric contraction).

## Points to note

Following finger injury several things can affect grip. Joint stiffness may limit the ability to bend the fingers sufficiently to form the grip shape, strength may be poor reducing grip force and/or time and skin sensation may be poor so you are unable to feel the object being gripped and judge appropriate force. To target each of these scenarios use the greatest variety of grips possible.

## Exercise 11.13 Resisted wrist abduction/adduction

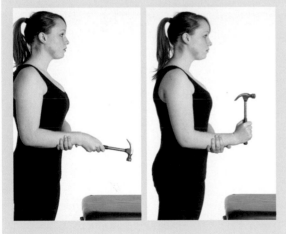

## Aims and usage

To re-strengthen the side-to-side (chopping) action of the wrist

## Starting position and instructions

Begin with your client standing facing a table and gripping a bar or small hammer by the handle, head up. Ensure they keep their elbow in its mid position with their thumb up and that they tuck their forearm into their side. Moving just their wrist, have them tip the hammer forwards and backwards as far as possible. Next, they should place the hammer head down and perform the same action, moving the hammer head in line with their forearm, forwards and backwards.

## Variations

Vary the speed of movement (rate) and amount of movement (range) to alter stress on the wrist.

## Points to note

• Where your client's wrist is very stiff, have them perform abduction/adduction closed chain stretch on table (Exercise 11.10) prior to doing this exercise.
• Holding a longer bar or gripping the hammer towards the end of the handle increases the leverage effect and makes the action harder

# LOW BACK AND PELVIS

# 12

## ANATOMY REFRESHER

### OVERVIEW

The spine is divided into cervical (neck), thoracic (mid) and lumbar (lower) regions, with the sacrum and coccyx forming the rudiments of your tail. The spinal column is made up of 33 individual bones (the vertebrae). Each vertebra is numbered to show its position. Cervical vertebra numbers begin with 'C', thoracic 'T', lumbar 'L' and sacral 'S', so, for example, the second cervical vertebra counting down from the head is C2, and the fourth C4. The last lumber vertebra is L5 (rather than L1) because the numbering system begins at the head each time (*see* Figure 12.1).

The lumbar vertebrae are large, strong bones covered with powerful muscles. They do not attach to the ribs, but their movements are intimately linked to those of the pelvis. The upper portion of the lumbar spine, L1 and L2, moves with the thoracic spine, especially during shoulder blade and ribcage movements. The lower lumbar vertebrae, L3, L4 and L5, move closely with the pelvis so that this combined region is often referred to as the lumbopelvis.

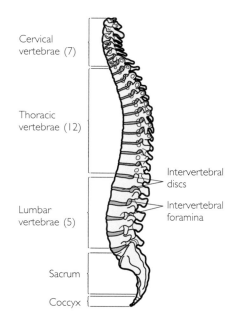

Cervical vertebrae (7)

Thoracic vertebrae (12)

Intervertebral discs

Intervertebral foramina

Lumbar vertebrae (5)

Sacrum

Coccyx

**Figure 12.1** The spinal vertebrae

### Keypoint

Vertebrae are numbered from the head down, with C1 just below the head and C7 between the shoulders.

## THE SPINAL SEGMENT

Each pair of spinal bones together forms a single unit called a *spinal segment* (*see* Figure 12.2). The two bones are separated by a spongy disc attached to the flat part of the bone. At the back of the vertebra the bone is extended to form two small joints called *facets*. From above it can be seen that the back of the spinal bone forms a hollow arch through which runs the spinal cord carrying messages from the brain to the legs and arms.

Gym users tend to talk about whole spine movements, bending and straightening, often not realising that segments of the spine can move relative to each other. Instructors look at specific segments of motion, for example, during an overhead shoulder exercise, the thoracic spine may be flattening while the lumbar spine curves excessively. Therapists look in even closer detail at the individual spinal segments. They are interested in the motion between L5/L4 relative to that of L4/L3, for example. Motion of an individual spinal segment can be important because stiffness in one segment following injury may cause a neighbouring segment to move excessively (known as 'compensatory hypermobility'), causing pain. The answer to this is to make the stiff segment move more so that the lax segment can move less. A physiotherapist often uses joint manipulation to release a stiff spinal segment and then exercise therapy to re-educate the muscles supporting the lax segment.

### Keypoint

Look closer at spinal movements. Notice movement of (i) the whole spine, (ii) regions of the spine relative to each other, and (iii) individual spinal segments.

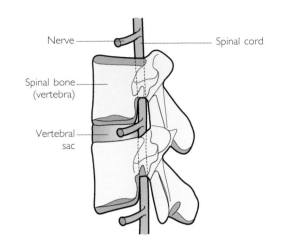

**Figure 12.2** A spinal segment

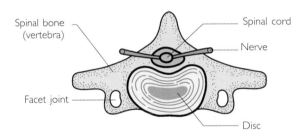

**Figure 12.3** The spinal bone carries the spinal cord

## SACRUM AND PELVIS

Below the lumbar vertebrae are the remnants of our tail. The sacrum is a triangular shaped bone which attaches at the sides to the pelvis, while the coccyx forms a thin, pointed tip to the end of the spine (*see* Figure 12.1). Both of these regions are important in terms of injury, especially during pregnancy and childbirth.

The joint between the sacrum and the pelvis (sacroiliac joint, *see* Figure 12.4) is filled with fibrous material and normally gives little

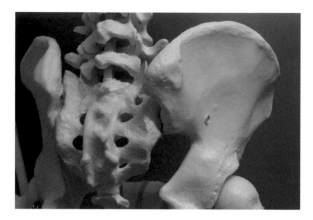

**Figure 12.4** The sacroiliac joint

movement. During childbirth, however, the fibrous material softens and the joint moves to allow the pelvis to expand to facilitate childbirth.

The coccyx again becomes more mobile in this period and can give problems. In addition, in the lean individual the coccyx is easily damaged by sitting or falling backwards directly onto a hard floor (*see* Figure 12.2). When performing exercise lying down it is important that clients use a mat to protect the coccyx from pressure. Particularly lean subjects may require a folded towel placed beneath the region additionally.

### Keypoint

The sacroiliac joint joins the sacrum to the pelvis. It is often painful during pregnancy and following childbirth.

## SPINAL CURVES

Although the spinal vertebrae stand one on top of each other, the column they make is not straight. Instead, the spine forms an 'S' curve. There are two inward curves in the lower back and neck, while the thoracic spine curves gently outwards. The inward curves are called the 'lumbar lordosis' and 'cervical lordosis', while the outward curve is the 'thoracic kyphosis'. When a client lies down on a bench, it is often necessary to support the curves with a rolled towel or pad to make them feel more comfortable, especially where they are suffering from low back or neck pain. In addition, the curves may increase or reduce in clients with these conditions, as a result of stiffness or muscle spasm. Restoration of the spinal curves is therefore an important aim of exercise therapy for this region.

The trunk forms a drum shape with the spine at the back. The spinal muscles (erector spinae) are close to the spinal bones, but the abdominal muscles (rectus abdominis, external oblique and internal oblique) also have an important effect on the spine. Even though they are positioned at the front of the body they are able to both move and support (stabilise) the spine.

## MOVEMENTS

Excessive movement in the lumbar spine can occur without us noticing. If a person bends forward to touch their toes or backward to look at the ceiling, the movement is obvious. But there is another way that the lumbar spine can move which is more subtle. The pelvis is connected directly to the lumbar spine (*see* Figure 12.5) and in turn balances rather like a seesaw on the hip joints. Because it is balanced, the pelvis can tilt forwards and backwards. As it tilts, the pelvis pulls the spine with it. If the pelvis tips down (*see* Figure 12.5a), the arch in the lumbar spine increases in a way equivalent to moving the spine backwards into 'extension'. When the pelvis tilts up (*see* Figure 12.5c), the lumbar curve is flattened, and the movement in the lumbar spine is equivalent to 'flexion', or forward bending.

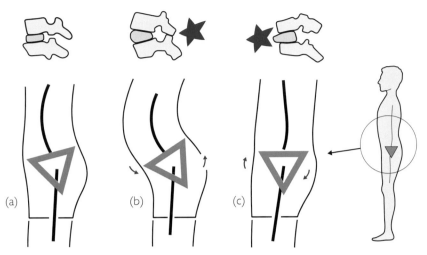

**Figure 12.5** Pelvic movement: (a) forward tilting – lower back hollow; (b) normal – lower back neutral; (c) backward tilting – lower back flattens

If the movement of the pelvis is excessive, the spine in turn is pulled to its end-range, stressing the spinal tissues. Note that it is only the lumbar spine which is moving. The rest of the spine remains largely unchanged, so the person is still standing upright.

---

**Keypoint**

Movement of the pelvis directly affects the lumbar spine.

---

The ratio between movement of the lumbar spine on the pelvis, and movement of the pelvis on the hip joints is important, and this combined motion of both body segments is called the 'lumbopelvic rhythm'. When you bend forwards to reach down to a desk from standing, for example, you have a choice. You could lock your pelvis and bend only from the spine (*see* Figure 12.6a), second

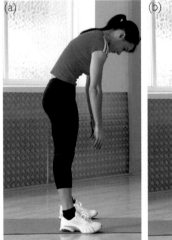
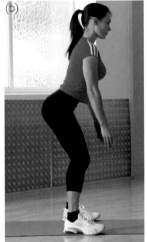

**Figure 12.6** Bending forward: (a) From the spine; (b) from the hips

you could keep your spine stiff and move from your hip alone (*see* Figure 12.6b) or third you could combine the two movements and move from both your hips and spine. The third motion is actually the one which places less stress on the body.

155

By moving the pelvis on the hips, the requirement for spine bending (lumbar flexion) is reduced and so the lumbar discs are protected. If, however, you keep your spine completely rigid, the lumbar muscles are overworked and can go into spasm, causing muscle pain. Allowing the spine to bend and then straightening the muscles, contracting and then relaxing is more healthy. Ideally, you should use twice as much pelvic movement as lumbar movement in everyday activities (a lumbopelvic ratio of 1:2). Commonly, however, people often forget to move from their pelvis and so the lumbar spine does most of the work, giving a lumbopelvic ratio of 3:1 with the pelvis moving only when the lumbar spine has moved to its end-range. It is important that you observe a client performing exercise very closely. Think about quality of movement rather than quantity. If a client is bending forward and performing a certain range of motion, analyse *where* that motion is coming from.

---

### Keypoint

When bending forward the ratio of lumbar movement (flexion) to pelvic movement (anterior tilt) is called the lumbopelvic rhythm. Ideally this should be 1:2 when bending for objects at table height.

---

## NEUTRAL POSITION

We have seen that as we move the spine the alignment of the spinal bones and tissues changes. For example, as we flex forwards the facet joints open and the tissues on the back of the spine stretch while those on the front relax. At the same time the pressure within the spinal discs increases. This combination of pressure and stretch, if repeated over and over again, can damage the spinal tissues.

If, however, we align the spinal tissues so the spine is upright and the lumbar region is comfortably curved, the spinal tissues are now at their normal length and the pressure within the discs is lowered. We call this normal alignment of the spine the 'neutral position' (*see* Figure 12.5b). It is one of the safest postures for the spine, and is a good starting point for spinal exercise practice.

To find your own neutral position, stand with your back to a wall. Your buttocks and shoulders should touch the wall. Place the flat of your hand between the wall and the small of your back. Try to tilt your pelvis so you flatten your back and then tilt your pelvis the other way so you increase the hollow in the lower back. Your neutral position (and it is slightly different for each person) is halfway between the flat and hollow positions.

You should just be able to place the flat of your hand between your back and the wall. If you can only place your fingers through, your back is too flat; if your whole hand up to your wrist can pass through the space, your back is too hollow.

---

### Keypoint

In the neutral position the spine is correctly aligned and the spinal tissues are held at the right length.

---

To find neutral position on a client or training partner, have them stand up against a wall with their hands out in front, arms straight (standing press-up position). Stand behind them (*see* Figure

12.7) side-on, and with their permission reach your left forearm around their waist, placing it across their waistband. Press your left shoulder against the back of their ribcage and the flat of your right hand over their sacrum. Their upper body is effectively fixed by their hands on the wall (they must keep their arms straight) and your left shoulder pressing against the back of their ribcage. Your left hand monitors the front of their pelvis and your right the back (sacrum). Using this position you can help them to tilt their pelvis with your hands guiding or 'cueing' the movement. Using touch in this fashion to give feedback is called tactile cueing and is an effective way of teaching, often cutting down many frustrating hours of practice for a client. Initially, simply tilt the pelvis, trying to encourage full range movement, and then stop in the neutral position.

## Keypoint

Use tactile cueing with a client to help them find neutral position of the lumbar spine.

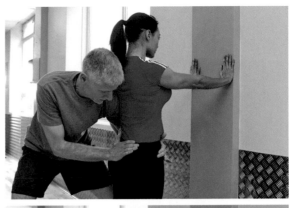

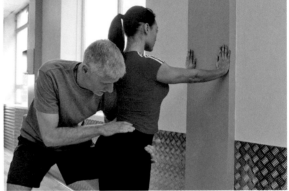

**Figure 12.7** Finding neutral pelvic position on a client

## Exercise 12.1 Abdominal hollowing in lying using belt

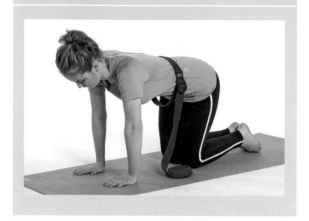

### Aims and usage

To begin retraining the abdominal hollowing action in cases of poor muscle control

### Starting position and instructions

Begin with your client kneeling with their hands directly beneath their shoulders and knees directly beneath the hips (in box position). Place a webbing belt around your client's waist between the pelvis and umbilicus. Have them relax their abdominal muscles and tighten the belt to just touch the skin surface. Have them focus their attention on the abdominal region and gently draw the abdominal wall inwards, away from the belt. They should hold the position for 3–5 seconds and then relax.

### Variations

• Have your client perform a pelvic floor contraction prior to abdominal hollowing. They should use the sensation of the pelvic floor contraction in the perineum to spread upwards towards the lower abdominal muscles.

• To avoid holding the breath, ask your client to count out loud from one to ten during the abdominal hollowing action.

### Points to note

The action must be an isolated abdominal movement without expanding the chest or holding the breath. No spinal movement (rounding or arching) should occur.

## Exercise 12.2 Abdominal hollowing sitting

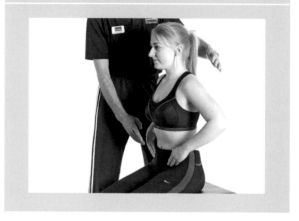

### Aims and usage

To rehearse the abdominal hollowing action in a functional sitting position

### Starting position and instructions

Begin with your client sitting on a low gym bench in an upright position (do not allow them to slouch). Have them place their thumbs beneath their trouser/shorts waistband and put the band forwards away from their skin about 1cm. Have them keep their chest and shoulders still, and draw their abdominal wall inwards away from their waistband. They should hold the position for 3–5 seconds and then repeat.

## Variations

• If you find your client sways as they perform this exercise, have them sit on a bench with their back against a wall.

• If you find your client is holding his/her breath, have them count out loud from one to ten as they perform the hollowing action.

## Points to note

This is an important exercise, as abdominal hollowing begins the process of re-establishing core stability. Stability is important in lifting and bending actions, but equally important in sitting actions. Sitting and reaching forward to lift a heavy book or folder off a tabletop, for example, can place severe stress on the lower back if muscular stability is poor.

---

### Exercise 12.3 Pelvic tilt against wall

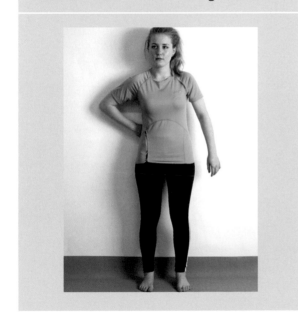

### Aims and usage

To strengthen and shorten the abdominal muscles and flatten the lumbar lordosis

### Starting position and instructions

Begin with your client standing with their back against a wall, feet slightly forwards enabling them to take their bodyweight back onto the wall (they should fall back onto the wall). Have them tighten their abdominal muscles and press the curve of their back (lumbar lordosis) flat onto the wall. They should hold this position for 5–10 seconds, breathing normally, and then release.

### Variations

• If the curve in your client's low back is quite deep (lordotic posture), place a folded towel between their back and the wall and have them press against that.

• Place your hand between the wall and your client's back to give them tactile feedback as they progress through the exercise.

### Points to note

To flatten the back against the wall two movements occur. The pelvis tips backwards (posterior pelvic tilt) and the low back flattens (lumbar flexion). To achieve a flat back this exercise is doing two things: shortening and strengthening the abdominal muscles and stretching the hip flexor muscles. If your client's hip flexors are very tight and their abdominals long and weak, have them perform a hip flexor stretch prior to doing this exercise to make the movement more obtainable.

## Exercise 12.4 Hip hitch

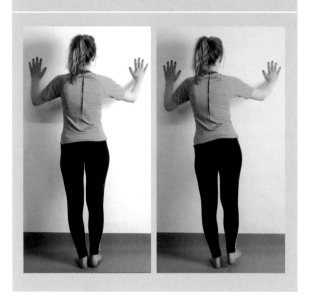

### Aims and usage
To begin restoring hip and pelvic control when standing

### Starting position and instructions
Begin with your client standing facing a wall with their hands flat on the wall. Keeping their legs straight, they should hitch one hip upwards, drawing the rim of their pelvis (iliac crest) closer to their lower ribs. Have them hold the position for 3–5 seconds and then release. Your client should perform the exercise on both sides of the body.

### Variations
• Have your client place their left foot on a low block to lower their pelvis to the right. They should hitch the right hip from this position for a greater motion range.

• Have them perform the exercise freestanding to improve standing balance.

### Points to note
By hitching (moving) the right leg, you are working the hip abductor muscles on the left and the trunk side flexors on the right.

## Exercise 12.5 Supported side bend

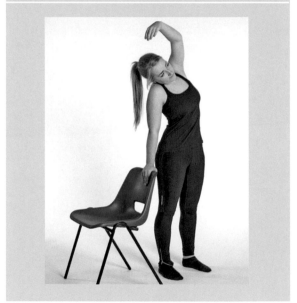

### Aims and usage
To lengthen the trunk side flexors in a supported starting position

### Starting position and instructions
Begin with your client standing side-on to a high bench, chair back or table (a kitchen work surface is ideal). Have your client stand with their feet shoulder-width apart and place their right hand on the tabletop. Ask them to bend their body to

the right (spinal side flexion), reaching their left hand overhead to try to touch their ear with the side of their upper arm. They should then take their bodyweight through their left hand onto the tabletop, and hold the stretched position for 3–5 seconds. Reverse the action, having them reach with their right hand and support with their left.

## Variations

• If there is no table or bench available, have your client place their left hand onto the rim of their pelvis to take some of the weight.

• To convert this exercise from a stretch to a strengthening exercise have your client place their hands behind their neck and perform the side-bend action. As they bend they're holding their bodyweight with eccentric (lowering body) and then isometric (holding at the bottom of movement) muscle activity.

## Points to note

This action stretches the trunk side flexors (obliques and quadratus lumborum) by performing a side-bend action. Reaching the arm overhead also stretches the latissimus dorsi and thoracolumbar fascia.

### Clinical scenario – acute low back pain

Acute low back pain often affects several structures including discs, spinal joints and soft tissues. Inflammation and muscle spasm often result and these can be a major cause of pain. Physiotherapy is the first choice of treatment, but exercise therapy is key as pain begins to subside. Spinal rotation using chair (Exercise 12.17) can be a useful technique to release muscle spasm in the low back. Have your client gradually ease into the position and expect it to take 5–10 reps before their movement range increases. Often back pain occurs through repeated flexion (bending) actions, so extension (arching) can be used to compensate and relieve pain. Lying spinal extension (Exercise 12.13) can be usefully modified. Rather than your client using their back muscles to pull them into extension (active extension), they place their arms on the floor in a press-up position and use their arms to press them into extension (passive extension), keeping their hips on the floor and their back muscles as relaxed as possible. Because pain often occurs to one side more than the other, you may notice that your client's spine bends to one side (known as 'scoliosis'). Use hip shift against wall (Exercise 12.16) to stretch the tighter side or supported side bend (Exercise 12.5) to stretch and open out the side of your client's trunk. In all cases when using exercise therapy for low back pain the first few reps may feel tight and sore for your client, but this should then ease as they work through the reps. The golden rule is for your client never to work through increasing pain. If their back hurts as they perform an exercise, they should wait for it to ease. If it does not ease, they should stop after a maximum of 8–10 reps. However, if the pain gets worse, have them stop immediately and rest until the pain goes before trying again.

## Exercise 12.6 Kneeling weight shift

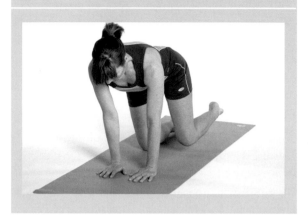

### Aims and usage

To begin rotary control in core stability

### Starting position and instructions

Begin with your client kneeling in the box position with their hands directly below their shoulders and knees directly below their hips. Have them gently tighten their abdominal muscles to suck them in a little (abdominal hollowing). They then move their pelvis to the right, keeping their hips horizontal until their left knee begins to lift from the floor (unloading). Have them hold this position for 2–3 seconds and then move it to the left to unload their right knee.

### Variations

• So that your client gets greater feedback about their hip position, have them place a hardback book on their pelvis (sacral area) and as they move they should aim to keep the book horizontal to prevent it sliding off.
• When your client unloads their knee have them hold it off the ground by 1cm and then move it forwards and backwards (hip flexion/

extension) for 5 reps and then side to side (hip abduction/adduction) for 5 reps.

### Points to note

The focus of this exercise is control rather than the quantity of movement obtained. Have your client begin with small, controlled movements of the leg and build up the movement range as they are able to move without losing alignment of their pelvis and lumbar spine.

## Exercise 12.7 Kneeling leg lift

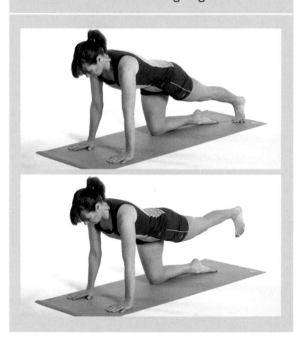

### Aims and usage

To offer an increased challenge to the core stability system

### Starting position and instructions

Begin with your client kneeling in the box position

with their hands directly below their shoulders and knees directly below their hips. Ensure that their spine is in a neutral position with a slight hollow in the low back (lumbar lordosis). Have them gently draw their abdominal muscles inwards (abdominal hollowing). Holding this spinal alignment, they then lift their left leg backwards to touch their left toes onto the floor behind them. They should hold this position for 2–3 seconds and then bring their leg back to the kneeling position and reverse the action, lifting their right leg.

## Variations

•  To increase the workload, have your client lift their leg up to the horizontal position rather than keeping their toes resting on the floor.
•  As a variation, rather than your client taking their leg back to its bent position in kneeling, have them keep it straight with their toes to the floor before lifting their straight leg again.

## Points to note

Although your client is focused on leg movement throughout this exercise, they should also be mindful of their spinal position. Ensure that they maintain spinal alignment and do not overly hollow their back (lordotic position), overly round it (flat back), or dip their pelvis to one side, which causes the spine to twist.

## Exercise 12.8 Kneeling leg and arm lift

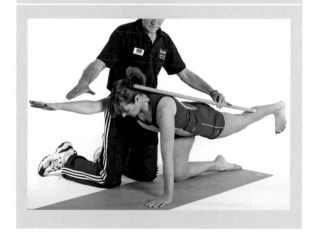

## Aims and usage

To offer an advanced challenge to the core stability system

## Starting position and instructions

Begin with your client kneeling in the box position with their hands directly below their shoulders and knees directly below their hips. Ensure that their spine is in a neutral position with a slight hollow in the low back (lumbar lordosis). Have them gently draw their abdominal muscles inwards (abdominal hollowing). Holding this spinal alignment, they should lift their left leg backwards to the horizontal position, and their right arm forwards to the horizontal. Have them hold this position for 2–3 seconds and then bring their leg and arm back to the kneeling position and reverse the action, lifting their right leg and left arm.

## Variations

•  To reduce loading with this exercise, have your client stretch both their leg and arm to floor level only. Advise them to keep their toes and fingertips on the floor surface for support and balance.
•  To progress from this lift, have them lift their leg to the horizontal but keep their hand on the floor and vice versa.

## Points to note

When you lift the opposite arm and leg there is a rotation stress (torsion) imposed on the spine. The aim of this exercise is to support the trunk against this stress and maintain optimal spinal alignment, keeping both the shoulders and hips level in a horizontal plane.

---

### Exercise 12.9 Trunk curl

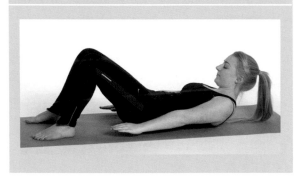

### Aims and usage

To shorten and strengthen the abdominal muscles

### Starting position and instructions

Begin with your client lying on the floor with their knees bent and hands by their sides. They should tuck their chin in (cervical flexion) and roll through their spine to look towards their hips, lifting just their shoulder blades from the floor. At the same time they should reach their hands forwards along the floor surface. Have them hold the maximum reach (full spinal flexion) for 3–5 seconds, breathing normally and then releasing.

### Variations

• Where your client's abdominal muscles are lengthened and they find this exercise especially difficult, have them begin with their shoulders raised on a wedge (one large cushion with a smaller one on top) to partially flex their trunk. Have them perform just the last part of the action, lifting their trunk by 1–2cm from the wedge to perform an inner range trunk curl. Help them lift forwards (assisted trunk flexion) before they lower themselves under their own muscle power (eccentric action).

### Points to note

The aim of this exercise is to flex the trunk using a curling action rather than lift the trunk from the ground. The lower back should stay on the ground throughout the action.

---

### Exercise 12.10 Lying pelvic tilt

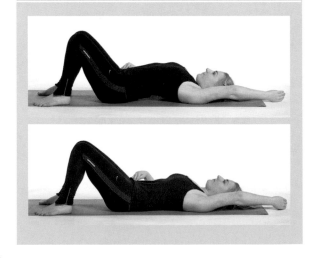

### Aims and usage

To rehearse the pelvic tilting action in a gravity-eliminated starting position

## Starting position and instructions

Begin with your client lying on the floor with their knees bent and arms relaxed, perhaps with hands on their hips, fingertips resting on their abdomen. Ask them to tighten their abdominal muscles and press their back flat against the floor and then continue the movement to lift their tailbone off the floor (lumbar flexion). Reverse the action, asking them to tighten their back muscles to increase the arch of the lower back (lumbar extension). Throughout the movements they should keep their buttocks on the floor.

## Variations

• This is often a difficult skill to master, so move your client's pelvis for them for 2–3 reps (passive movement) and then they can follow the action with their muscle strength (assisted movement).

• Increase the work intensity on the abdominal muscles by having your client pause in the inward position with their tailbone off the ground for 5 seconds (inner range hold).

## Points to note

Have your client use their hands on their lower abdomen to monitor the movement, feeling their pelvis move.

---

## Exercise 12.11 Lying knee roll

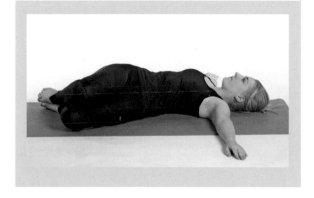

### Aims and usage

To release tension in the lower spine

### Starting position and instructions

Begin with your client lying on the floor with their knees bent to 90 degrees, hips to 45 degrees and feet flat. Have them take their arms out to the side, roughly level with their shoulders (80–90-degree abduction). Keeping their feet on the floor, they should then twist (rotate) their spine to lower their knee down to the floor on one side of their body. They should pause and then lift their knees back to the starting position before lowering them to the floor on the other side of their body.

### Variations

• Where your client is unable to comfortably lower their knees all the way to the floor, place cushions or yoga blocks on the floor at knee level. They can then lower their knees to the cushions rather than the floor (reduced range of motion).

• Have your client keep their left leg straight and rotate the spine to the left, placing their right knee onto the floor on the left side of their body to perform a lying single bent leg twist. Have them repeat the action with their right leg straight and left bent. By keeping one leg straight, their bent knee lowers further to the ground, emphasising *stretch* of the spine and trunk rotator muscles.

• Have them bend their hips and knees to 90 degrees so their knees lie directly above their hips and their feet are completely lifted from the floor. They should then lower their knees slowly to the floor, not allowing them to drop, to perform a crunch roll exercise. By taking the full leg weight, the resistance to movement is greater, emphasising the *strength* of the trunk rotator muscles.

## Points to note

This action combines a stretch of the spine and trunk rotator muscles with a stretch of the same body part. The action must be controlled. If the legs are allowed to fall to the floor uncontrolled, the stress on the spine is excessive and potentially dangerous.

### Clinical scenario – chronic low back pain

It is common for people to suffer from low back pain for years. Often this can be traced back to a single seemingly innocent incident which hurt. Your client rested and the pain eased, but it keeps coming back if they sit for a long time, for example, while driving or after a bout of gardening or simply picking up their kids. This is chronic low back pain and the single most important aspect of its treatment is exercise therapy. The reason that back pain recurs is twofold: alignment and back fitness. First, after the initial bout of pain alignment changes. The curve in the low back can flatten or the back can be pulled to the side slightly. Although you may not notice these changes it means that any loading placed on the back, for example through work, will be uneven, over-stressing some structures and under-working others. Alignment is important for a second reason. Much of our time nowadays is spent on computers or driving and these are flexion (bending) movements. Put simply, excessive flexion tightens the front of the body and over stretches the back, so you literally start to become chair shaped, unable to stand up straight. When you have back pain you cannot move much or exercise and as a result your muscles become weaker and your spine stiffens. Because this is associated with pain it is common for people to accept this as a normal part of ageing and not to try to exercise. However, exercise is the key to recovery with this condition, if used correctly.

Begin addressing alignment using pelvic tilt against a wall (Exercise 12.3) to identify the neutral position of your client's low back (depth of the curve) and to increase local mobility. Use abdominal hollowing lying (Exercise 12.1) and/or sitting (Exercise 12.2) to begin redeveloping muscle strength to support the back (core stability) and use lying knee roll (Exercise 12.11) to reduce stiffness. This is especially useful to do in the evening when your client gets back from work if their job involves sitting for a long time. The kneeling leg lift (Exercise 12.7) and kneeling leg and arm lift (Exercise 12.8, also called the 'bird dog') works core stability well by using the leverage effects of the limbs to overload the trunk muscles back and front. The hip hinge (Exercise 12.12) begins the process of transferring the good alignment your client has begun to learn into bending and eventually lifting actions.

## Exercise 12.12 Hip hinge

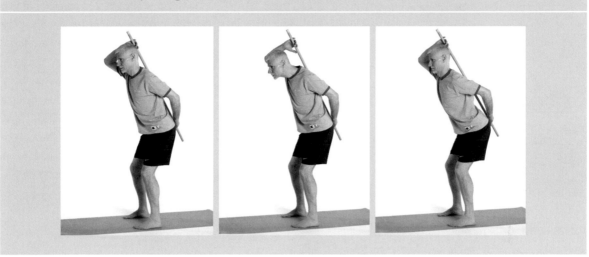

### Aims and usage
To restore correct lumbopelvic rhythm

### Starting position and instructions
Begin with your client standing with their feet hip-width apart. Place a pole (broom handle) along the length of their spine and have them reach overhead with one hand to grasp the top of the pole, and behind their back with the other hand to grasp the bottom of the pole. Their tailbone (sacrum), shoulders and head should be in contact with the stick. They should then slightly bend their knees to unlock them and tip their trunk forward, keeping it straight and moving from their hips (anterior pelvic tilt). Ensure they stop when their body is angled to 45 degrees and then return to the upright position.

### Variations
• Vary your client's range of motion. Have them angle the trunk to 20, 45 and then 90 degrees, each time pausing in the angled position for 2–3 seconds before returning.
• Instead of using the stick to monitor your client's spinal position, have them place their hands behind their back (low resistance) or behind their head (higher resistance).

### Points to note
The aim of this exercise is to keep the spine straight as you bend forwards using anterior pelvis tilt. If you round the shoulders and bend the upper spine (thoracic spine flexion), the head moves away from the stick. If you bend the lower spine (lumbar spine flexion), the stick moves away from the sacrum. Finally, if you increase the depth of the lumbar curve (lordosis), the gap between the low back and the stick significantly increases.

167

## Exercise 12.13 Lying spinal extension

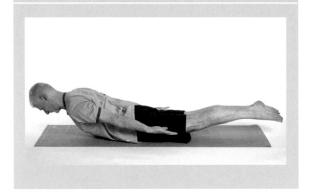

### Aims and usage
To strengthen the back and hip extensors to full inner range

### Starting position and instructions
Have your client lie on their front with their arms by their sides. Ask them to tighten their thigh muscles (quadriceps) and lift their legs so that their knees clear the floor by 5–10cm. At the same time they should reach their fingers to the outsides of their ankles and lift their chest so their breastbone (sternum) clears the floor also by 5–10cm. Have them hold the top position (inner range) and then lower under control.

### Variations
• To increase resistance, have your client place their hands behind their neck rather than at their sides.
• To slightly reduce resistance, have them lift one leg at a time.
• To further reduce resistance, have them bend their elbows and place their forearms flat on the floor to the sides of their chest (in assisted spinal extension). They should use their arms to assist the chest lift and keep their legs on the floor first. As they become stronger, encourage them to offer less assistance to the chest lift by pressing less with their arms and instead lifting one leg.

### Points to note
The aim of this action is to focus on spinal strength rather than movement range. The lift should be from the floor, but not too high. The combination of spinal extension and muscle shortening compresses the spine and a greater range of motion may be too stressful on the spinal facet joints where a client is recovering from injury.

## Exercise 12.14 Lying single/double leg lift

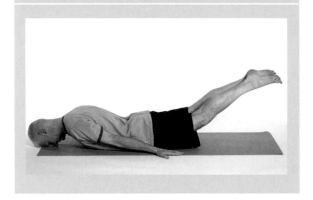

### Aims and usage
To strengthen the spinal and hip extensor muscles focusing on lumbar movement alone

### Starting position and instructions
Begin with your client lying on the floor with their hands by their sides, palms down. Have them tighten their thigh (quadriceps) muscles to straighten their legs and press down on the floor

with their hands and arms to lift their legs clear of the floor by 5–10cm. Have them hold the top position for 3–5 seconds, breathing normally and then lowering under control.

## Variations
• To reduce resistance, have your client lift one leg at a time.
• To increase the workload, have them hold their legs in the air for a longer period (5–10 seconds).

## Points to note
This action combines hip extension, anterior pelvic tilt and lumbar spine extension to work the hip and spinal extensors. To increase the work on the spinal extensors and reduce anterior pelvic tilt, have your client try to relax their buttock muscles (gluteals). To encourage this, ask them to focus on broadening across the buttocks and allowing their heels to move apart (in lateral hip rotation).

### Exercise 12.15 Standing dumbbell side bend

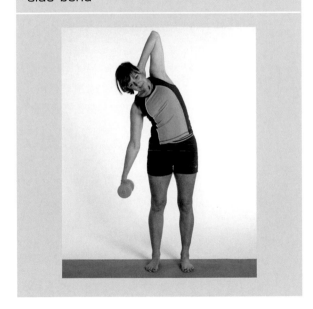

## Aims and usage
To strengthen the trunk side flexor muscles

## Starting position and instructions
Begin with your client standing with their feet shoulder-width apart. Have them hold a dumbbell or other weight in their right hand and place their left hand behind their head. They should then bend their trunk to the right allowing the dumbbell to reach down the side of their right leg to the outside of their knee. Have them pause in this lower position and then bend to the left, reaching their left elbow towards the floor. They should repeat the action, holding the weight in their left hand.

## Variations
• Rather than using a weight, have your client place both hands behind their neck (creating higher resistance) or at their sides (creating lower resistance) to perform a standing side bend exercise.

## Points to note
This action must be slow and controlled. A fast action builds momentum and may overly stress the lumbar tissues

## Exercise 12.16 Hip shift against wall

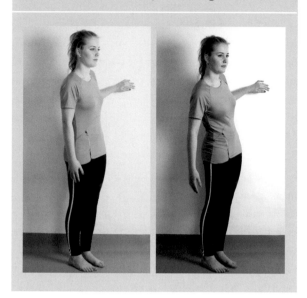

### Aims and usage

To correct a lateral spinal shift posture

### Starting position and instructions

Begin with your client standing left side-on to a wall with their feet together. Ask them to raise (abduct) their arm to shoulder level and place their forearm flat onto the wall. Have them press their hips in towards the wall, keeping their shoulders fixed and level, and then return to the standing position. They should repeat the action for between 5 and 10 repetitions.

### Variations

• To focus on static stretching, rather than performing multiple reps, have your client perform a single action and hold the inward full stretch position for 20–30 seconds.

• Where the spine is very stiff and there is little available movement, have them use their left hand to place overpressure on the rim of their pelvis. Have them press their hips in towards the wall a little further with each repetition.

### Points to note

This exercise is useful when your client has suffered an incident of low back pain which has left their pelvis out of alignment with their shoulders – a so-called 'shift' position. This may be caused by muscle spasm and/or pressure changes within the lumbar discs. If *repeated*, the exercise has a pumping action on the discs. If *held*, the focus moves to tight muscle, which is targeted through a continuous stretch.

## Exercise 12.17 Spinal rotation using chair

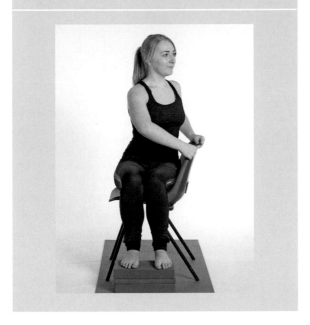

### Variations

• Use small, gentle, repeated pressures (pulsing) to encourage the spinal tissues to release.

• Rather than using pressure from the chair back, have your client place a pole (broom handle) across their shoulders and grasp each end. Use a slow, active rotation action, your client moving towards the chair back.

### Points to note

This action must be slow and controlled. Using a vigorous twisting movement builds momentum and can easily place high levels of stress on the delicate lumbar tissues.

### Aims and usage

To release spinal stiffness using self-applied passive rotation

### Starting position and instructions

Begin with your client sitting side-on to an upright chair (dining type or yoga chair) with their feet flat on the floor and hip-width apart. Have them turn towards the chair back and place their hands on the top of the back rest. They should move their elbows apart and sit upright, levelling their shoulders. Ask them to use their arms to provide overpressure to rotate their spine further towards the chair back. They should time the movement with their breath, pressing further as they exhale to encourage muscle relaxation.

# THORACIC SPINE // AND CHEST

**13**

## ANATOMY REFRESHER

The ribcage (thoracic cage) is egg shaped with the top narrow, broadening as it descends, and narrowing once more towards the bottom. The top and bottom of the 'egg' are cut off, with the top (above the first rib), called the *thoracic inlet*, leading to the neck, and the bottom (below the twelfth rib), called the *thoracic outlet*, leading to the abdomen.

The ribs connect to the thoracic spine at the back and the breastbone (sternum) at the front. There are twelve pairs of ribs, with numbers 1–10 attaching to the both the thoracic spine and sternum. Ribs 11 and 12 attach only to the thoracic spine, being free at their front end – hence their name 'floating ribs'

Anything to do with the ribs is known as 'costo' in medical terms, so the rib joint with the sternum is the sternocostal (SC) joint, that with the vertebra the costovertebral (CV) joint and that with the side bone (transverse process) of the vertebra the costotransverse (CT) joint (*see* Figure 13.1).

The intercostal muscles (there are three sets arranged in layers) lie between each adjacent pair of ribs and assist in breathing and raising and lowering the ribs during exercise. The breathing action involves four components:

(a)

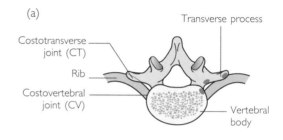

(b)

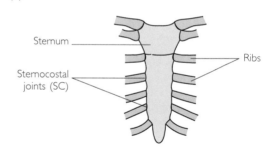

**Figure 13.1** The skeleton, showing the ribs and rib joints

1. **abdominal** (diagrammatic) breathing, where the abdominal wall expands outwards;
2. **costal** breathing, where the lower ribs flare out;
3. **sternal** breathing, where the breastbone lifts; and
4. **apical** breathing, where the top ribs and collar bone (clavicle) lift upwards.

Abdominal breathing is often referred to as *balloon breathing* as the abdominal wall forms a dome shape during inspiration to allow the diaphragm to descend. Costal breathing involves a sideways lifting of the ribs which are attached at the front and back, an action said to resemble lifting the handle of a bucket, hence the name *bucket handle breathing*. During sternal breathing, the sternum is lifted forwards, an action which is referred to as *pump handle breathing*.

For clients who have respiratory conditions such as asthma and bronchitis, for example, and also following injury to the ribcage, exercise to encourage lung expansion using each type of breathing is important.

---

### Exercise 13.1 Rib expansion using towel

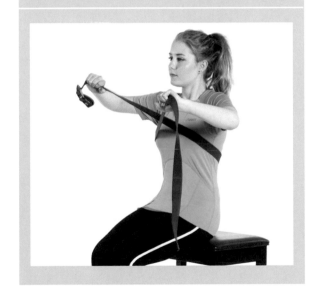

They should tighten the belt so that it grips their ribcage but does not prevent free movement. Ask them to take a deep breath in and press their ribs outwards against the belt – they should try to press equally with both sides of the ribcage, encouraging the injured side to move as much as the uninjured side. Ask them to relax and allow their breathing to normalise before repeating the action.

#### Variations
• Use a folded towel rather than a yoga belt.
• Rather than a belt or towel, have your client place the flat of their opposite hand (right hand for left side ribs) over the injured part of their ribcage. As they breath in they should try to expand the ribcage against their hand to perform *focused breathing*.

#### Aims and usage
To encourage ribcage expansion and intercostal muscle stretch following rib injury

#### Starting position and instructions
Begin with your client sitting on a gym bench. Place a belt around their chest. Have them hold the right end with their left hand and vice versa.

#### Points to note
The aim of this exercise is twofold: to encourage ribcage expansion (known as 'inspiratory volume') and symmetry between rib movement. Using the towel is useful for general expansion, but localising with the hand is better to focus on a single area that may be less mobile than a neighbouring region.

## Exercise 13.2 Overhead reach with stick

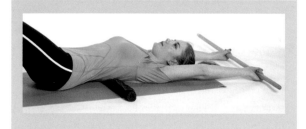

### Aims and usage

To combine ribcage expansion and thoracic spine extension

### Starting position and instructions

Begin with your client lying on the floor with a folded towel placed beneath their upper back (thoracic spine). Have them place the towel across their spine to act as a pivot for movement rather than lengthways along the spine. Ask them to bend their knees to flatten their lumbar spine towards the floor, keeping their feet flat. They should then reach overhead, keeping their arms straight and use the leverage of their arms to press their thoracic spine into extension over the towel. Have them hold the fully stretched position (maximum reach) for 3–5 seconds and then repeat.

### Variations

• Have your client grip a towel or pole between each hand to ensure that they move both arms equally and allow the weight of the towel to press their arms back further towards the ground when overhead.

• Have them remain in the overhead position and with each repetition bring the arms back slightly (10–15cm) and then press once more using a gentle pulsing stretch.

• Have them perform the exercise in sitting, ensuring that the spine remains well aligned and the lumbar region does not hyperextend.

### Points to note

It is important to separate thoracic spine extension from ribcage expansion. When your client is performing this exercise, ask them to try to breath relatively normally rather than simply taking a deep breath. They should not hold their breath, but rest between reps to allow their breathing to normalise. Breathing too deeply or holding the in-breath can cause you to take in too much air (hyperventilate) and feel dizzy.

## Exercise 13.3 Sitting sternal lift

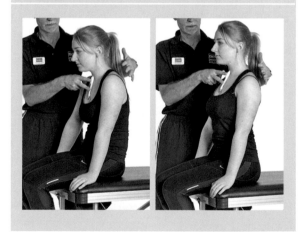

### Aims and usage

To develop control of active thoracic extension

### Starting position and instructions

Begin with your client sitting on a gym bench or firm chair with their feet and knees hip-width

174

apart and feet flat on the floor. Place the edge of a small, firm book (or use a yoga block) flat against your client's breastbone (sternum). In a relaxed and slouched position the book angles downwards. Keeping the book pressed firmly against the sternum, your client should draw their shoulder blades down and at the same time lift their sternum so the book points forwards and slightly upwards.

## Variations

• If your client finds holding the book awkward, monitor their sternal position with your fingertips and give feedback (tactile cueing) as they move.

• Have them perform the exercise with their back against a wall. As they draw their shoulder blades downwards, they should feel them sliding down the wall.

## Points to note

Where the thoracic spine is stiff or in cases of osteoporosis there is very little movement within the thoracic spine. However, the exercise is still helpful as the act of lifting the sternum and drawing the shoulder blades downwards helps to stretch the chest tissues and strengthen the postural shoulder muscles (scapular stabilisers).

---

## Exercise 13.4 Thoracic side bend

## Aims and usage

To open the ribcage at the side and laterally flex the thoracic spine

## Starting position and instructions

Begin with your client standing with their back against a wall and placing their hands behind

their neck. Have them focus on their breastbone (sternum), using it as their pivot point. Ask them to reach their left elbow down and their right upwards, keeping their sternum central rather than allowing it to tip to the side. Reverse the action to stretch the other side of their ribcage.

## Variations

• Where your client cannot easily place their hands behind their head, have them place the backs of their hands on their forehead instead.
• Rather than placing their hands on their head, place a stick across their shoulders and ask them to hold the ends of the stick.

## Points to note

This exercise is only effective if lateral flexion is isolated to the thoracic spine. To ensure this, your client' s sternum must not move from the midline. The action should be to rotate around the sternum, which acts as a pivot point. If the sternum moves to the side, lateral flexion of the lumbar spine is occurring (see photo).

## Exercise 13.5 Dumbbell flye on gym ball

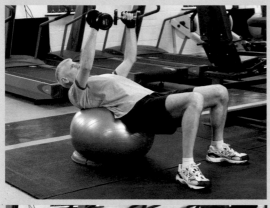

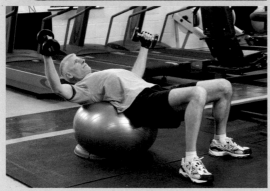

### Aims and usage

To expand the ribcage and work the chest musculature

### Starting position and instructions

Begin by having your client support their shoulders on a gym ball, feet wider than hip-width apart to aid whole body stability. Place a light (2–5kg) dumbbell in each of their hands. Have them begin with their hands together above their breastbone and elbows slightly bent. They should reach their arms out sideways and slightly upwards so that their hands finish in a horizontal line with their shoulders. Have them hold the fully stretched position for 1–2 seconds and then return to the starting position.

### Variations

- If your client's chest is very tight, have them begin performing the exercise without dumbbells to stretch their chest using arm weight alone.
- Kneel behind them and support their elbows with your cupped hands in the lowest part of the exercise – a technique called *spotting*.

### Points to note

This exercise combines stretch with strength. To focus on stretching, use light weights and a greater range of motion, asking your client to take their arms down as far as possible. For strength, use heavier weights and stop the arms just short of the fully stretched lower position.

## Exercise 13.6 Gym ball lat stretch

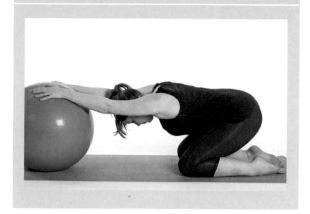

### Aims and usage

To extend the thoracic spine and stretch the shoulders

### Starting position and instructions

Begin with your client kneeling on a mat with a gym ball placed in front of them. Have them reach out to straighten their arms and place their hands on the top of the gym ball, keeping them shoulder-width apart. Ask them to sit slightly backwards and at the same time press their chest downwards, but to keep their head raised (extended). They should pause in the low position for 1–2 seconds and then repeat.

### Variations

• If you find your client's hands are too close together, have them grip a stick between their hands and press down on the gym ball with the stick.
• If your client finds kneeling painful, fold one or two towels and place them on the floor beneath their knees.

### Points to note

The aim of this exercise is to extend the thoracic spine and so open the chest. Keeping the head up encourages the upper thoracic spine to extend.

## Clinical scenario – ribcage injury

Ribcage injury is common in sport from a direct blow such as a knee in rugby, but may also occur with violent coughing episodes. Ribs may be cracked (fractured) and the intercostal muscles running between each pair of ribs torn. Remember also that the ribs have small joints at their ends, attaching at the front to the breastbone (sternum) and the back of the spine. As you breath, the ribs move apart and tilt upwards and forwards.

Any injury affecting the ribs normally presents as pain when breathing deeply, but it may also hurt as you twist your spine, pulling on the rib joints. Rib expansion using towel (Exercise 13.1) is useful to identify and correct stiffness on one side of the ribs and overhead reach with stick (Exercise 13.2) combines both rib expansion and thoracic extension. This is important because pain and tightness in the ribcage can cause a person to flatten their chest and hunch forwards, flexing their thoracic spine. The sitting sternal lift (Exercise 13.3) is useful to encourage thoracic extension. When one side of the ribcage is tighter than the other (asymmetry) thoracic side bend (Exercise 13.4) can help your client work through the imbalance.

## Exercise 13.7 Thoracic slump

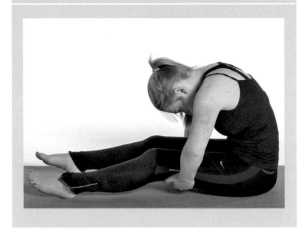

### Aims and usage

To stretch the nerves from the thoracic spine to the arms

### Starting position and instructions

Begin with your client sitting on the floor with their legs outstretched, knees unlocked by 20 degrees. Have them bend their spine, bringing their forehead towards their upper thighs. Have them hold this position for 1–2 seconds and then grip their hands behind their lower thighs. Again, they should hold the position for 1–2 seconds and then finally tighten their thigh muscles (quadriceps) to lock out their knees.

### Variations

• Place a very gentle pressure onto their head and upper spine to encourage the spinal bend.
• Have them perform the exercise on a bench and leave one leg bent over the bench side to perform a single leg thoracic slump.
• Have them rotate their spine, drawing their right shoulder downwards towards their left hip and vice versa.
• Rather than holding the stretch, ask them to move to the stretched point and then release, repeating this action 5–8 times. This method targets the movement of the nerve (neural mobility) rather than the nerve length.

### Points to note

This exercise is designed to stretch the nerves (neural stretch), which are very delicate. It is important that the action is performed very slowly with a gradual increase in movement range. Your client should feel an intense stretch, but not severe pain. Where pain occurs release the stretch by asking your client to unlock their knees and/or slightly straighten their spine.

## Exercise 13.8 Shoulder press

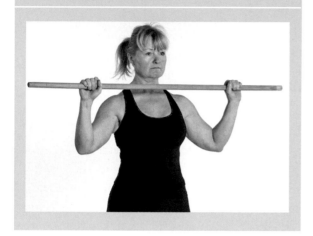

### Aims and usage
To strengthen the shoulder musculature while stabilising the trunk

### Starting position and instructions
Begin with your client standing with a light barbell or pole (broom handle) held in both hands, knuckles down. Have them place the bar on their upper chest, level with the top of their breastbone. They should then press the bar overhead, keeping it close to their face. Have them lock their arms out straight and then lower the bar under control back to the starting position.

### Variations
•   Where a heavier bar is used, your client should slightly flex their knees and extend them to create momentum in the bar to start the action. They should then straighten their legs as the bar passes overhead and flex them slightly to soften the bar's landing as they position it back to their breastbone.

•   This exercise can also be performed in sitting. In the sitting position it is important to maintain a neutral lumbar curve (lordosis) and not allow the lumbar spine to flatten or hollow excessively as this stresses the lumbar tissues.

•   Have them perform the exercise with the bar across their shoulders (press behind neck). As they press the bar upwards they should move their head forwards slightly, and as the bar descends draw their head back.

### Points to note
This exercise works the shoulder muscles, but maintaining good alignment of the trunk challenges the spinal stabilising muscles as the combined weight and leverage of the extended arms imposes high stresses on the spine.

# 14

# // HEAD AND NECK

## ANATOMY REFRESHER

We saw in Chapter 12 that the spine consists of 33 bones and the cervical (neck) region has seven, numbered C1 to C7. The C1 vertebrae forms a joint with the base of the skull while the C7 vertebra forms a joint with the first thoracic vertebra (T1). The cervical region is subdivided into two functional parts. The upper portion directly below the head is called the 'suboccipital region' (the *occiput* being the lower back portion of the skull). The C1 and C2 bones make up this region and they are intimately related to skull movements, especially nodding actions. The lower portion of the neck is called the 'lower cervical region' and takes in the bones C3 to C7. This region is more involved with twisting (rotation) and side bending (lateral flexion) actions.

## HEAD AND NECK POSTURE

We have seen that the spine forms an 'S' shape with inner curves (lordosis) in both the low back (lumbar lordosis) and neck (cervical lordosis). This alignment can be lost both as a result and cause of injury. Injury can cause a change in the relationship between one spinal bone to its neighbour, and muscle spasm can pull the whole neck out of alignment. Looking at a client's posture from behind, the contour of the shoulder muscles should be equal (symmetrical) on both sides and the head should be facing forwards rather than tilted to one side. Looking at the position of the centre of the head in relation to the midline, and the distance from the ear to the shoulder, gives us a good idea about postural changes (*see* Figure 14.1a). From the side (*see* Figure 14.1b) the ear should lie on the vertical posture line, that passes through the shoulder, and the eyes look straight ahead rather than up or down.

One of the most common postural changes in the neck is called a 'head held forwards' (HHF) posture, more commonly known as 'poking chin'. Normally the cervical lordosis should be quite shallow, with the curve going through the whole of the neck and the head held on the vertical posture line. If you imagine a long earring hanging down, the line should pass behind your client's collar bone. In the HHF posture this line passes in front of the collar bone through the upper chest. The head is too far forwards, but to get into this position the neck curve is not just increased, but it becomes uneven. The chin pokes forwards so that the curve close to the top of the neck (upper cervical region) bends back markedly into extension and the lower neck area (lower cervical

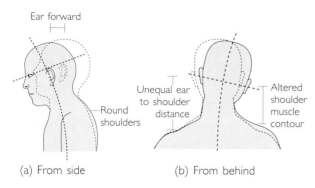

Ear forward

Round shoulders

(a) From side

Unequal ear to shoulder distance

Altered shoulder muscle contour

(b) From behind

**Figure 14.1** Checking postural change: (a) The centre of the head in relation to the midline; (b) the ear should lie on the vertical posture line

region) bends further forwards than normal into flexion. The result is a dramatic increase in pressure to the upper cervical region with the tissues becoming tight and painful. Stretching out this tight area and reversing the chin poke posture is a primary aim of treatment, and postural exercise for the head and neck is essential.

The poking chin posture gives upper cervical extension and lower cervical flexion. To correct this we can use an opposite action of upper cervical flexion and lower cervical extension (*see* Figure 14.2). This action is called a 'skull rock' and involves drawing the chin backwards as though forming a double chin and then looking downwards. Drawing the chin inwards (head retraction) flattens the neck moving the sub-occipital region into flexion and the lower cervical spine into extension – these two movements occurring because the 'S' shape of the neck is flattened. Looking downwards when the chin is tucked in to form the skull rock action increases the movement range.

Following injury on any part of the body both flexibility and strength are required. With the neck, however, it is common for clients to focus on flexibility in a bid to stretch out tight tissue, but to forget about strength. Following neck injury, both stability (cervical stability) and movement muscles should be worked initially to restore optimal posture and then to prepare individuals for higher stress actions in sports and daily life. Imagine a boxer or a rugby player in the scrum – if neck stability and strength is poor, re-injury is far more likely.

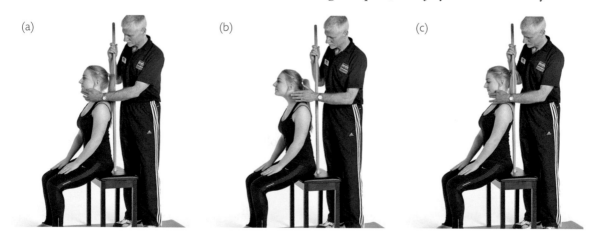

(a)  (b)  (c)

**Figure 14.2** Fixing postural change: (a) neutral posture; (b) head held forwards (HHF) posture; (c) retraction

## Exercise 14.1 Chin tuck

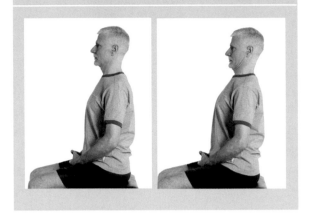

### Aims and usage
To perform upper cervical flexion coupled with lower cervical extension

### Starting position and instructions
Begin with your client sitting with their hands on their lap or forearms on a pillow resting on their lap to take the weight of their arms and relax their shoulder muscles. Have them draw their chin inwards as though trying to give themselves a double chin. Ask them to keep looking forwards rather than down, so their chin moves as though resting on a shelf. They should keep their shoulders relaxed and shouldn't shrug them. Have them hold the tucked chin position for 1–2 seconds and then release.

### Variations
• Have your client lace overpressure on their chin by pressing gently with the web space between their thumb and forefinger to encourage further inward (tucked) movement.
• Have your client resist the chin tuck action to strengthen the muscles pulling their chin in (the cervical retractors). Place a towel behind their head and have them hold each end of the towel with their hands. They should then press their head backwards against the resistance of the towel.

### Points to note
If your client's neck is very stiff and they have a very marked head forward posture, this exercise can be very difficult. To begin you may notice very little movement, but over time the movement range increases.

## Exercise 14.2 Skull rock standing back to wall

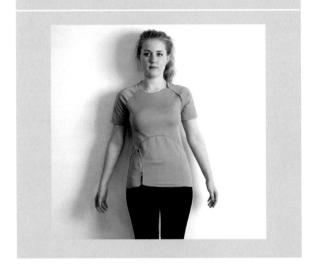

### Aims and usage
To rehearse the skull rock action in a self-monitored starting position

### Starting position and instructions
Begin with your client standing with their back to a wall. Have them place their feet slightly forwards so their bodyweight presses them back

onto the wall. They should feel the back of their head lightly touching the wall. Have them nod their head so that the part of their skull in contact with the wall (occiput) move upwards and downwards as though drawing the number 'one'.

## Variations
• If your client's head does not touch the wall, hold a book against the wall on which they rest their head.

• Have them perform the same action lying down with the back of their skull moving up and down on the floor.

## Points to note
Initially your client may feel very little movement, perhaps only 1cm. As their movement range increases, however, they should be able to move their head further and the number 'one' they are drawing becomes longer.

### Exercise 14.3 Isometric neck squeeze

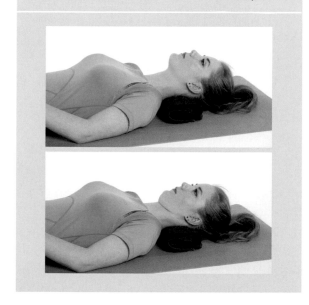

## Aims and usage
To strengthen the cervical retractor muscles

## Starting position and instructions
Begin with your client lying on the floor with their knees bent. Place a small rolled towel beneath the curve of their neck. Have them tuck their chin in to press their neck against the towel, trying to flatten out the cervical curve. They should hold the inner (towel compressed) position for 2–5 seconds and then release.

## Variations
• Physiotherapists often use a pressure bio-feedback unit when performing this exercise. This machine shows the exact pressure the client is applying when pressing the neck backwards, enabling you to monitor the amount of neck retraction.
• You may use a partially inflated long balloon in place of the towel.

## Points to note
The aim of this exercise is to improve the endurance of the neck retractor muscles. As the action becomes easier over time, increase the amount of time your client holds the towel compression up to 20–30 seconds rather than having them press harder. When holding for a prolonged period make sure that your client breathes normally and does not hold their breath.

## Exercise 14.4 Neck side flexion using band

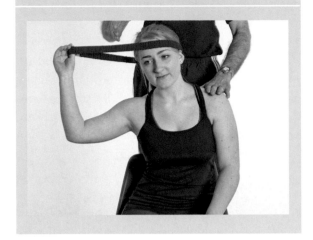

### Aims and usage

To work the neck side flexor muscles against resistance

### Starting position and instructions

Begin with your client sitting holding a loop of resistance band in their right hand. Hook the band around their head and have them hold their hand up to the right side of their head to take the slack from the band. They should tip their head to the left side (left lateral flexion), tightening the band. Have them hold the full position for 3–5 seconds and then release. Reverse the action, your client holding the band with their left hand and tipping their head to the right.

### Variations

• Rather than have your client holding the band, tie it securely to a gym machine or piece of furniture.
• If you have no band available, you can use manual resistance instead either from your or your client's hand.

### Points to note

As your client returns their head to the starting position, ensure they control the movement. Do not allow the resistance band to pull their head rapidly as this can excessively stress the cervical spine.

## Exercise 14.5 Cervical rotation with overpressure

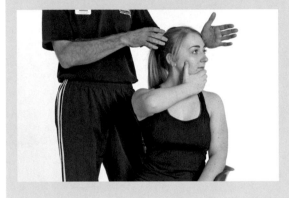

### Aims and usage

To increase rotation motion range at the neck

### Starting position and instructions

Begin with your client sitting upright with their feet flat on the floor. Ensure that their spine is correctly aligned with a neutral lumbar lordosis (neither excessively hollow or flat) and a neutral cervical lordosis (no poking chin). Have them turn their head to the left. When they get to their end-range, ask them to place their right hand onto the angle of their right jaw and gently press their head further into the rotation range. They should pause in the new end-range for 2–3 seconds and then slowly release. Repeat the action, this time turning to the right.

## Variations

• At end-range instead of holding the position, have your client use a gentle pulsing action, pressing and releasing. The movement with each pulse should be no more than 0.5cm and force only 5–10 per cent of maximum.

• Have your client perform the action sitting with their back to a wall and aim to keep their head the same distance from the wall as they turn. Do not allow them to let their head move forwards (protraction) or backwards (retraction) relative to the wall.

## Points to note

The aim of this action is to increase motion range while maintaining optimal head, neck and shoulder alignment. Ensure that your client does not allow their chin to poke forwards as they turn. In addition, ensure they keep their shoulder blades down, avoiding any shrugging (shoulder elevation) action.

---

### Exercise 14.6 Fist traction

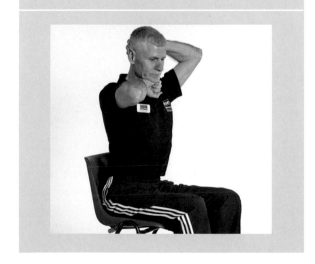

## Aims and usage

To induce focused traction to the upper cervical spine

## Starting position and instructions

Begin with your client sitting with their spine optimally aligned. Have them place their right fist thumb-side down (forearm pronation) between the top of their breastbone (sternum) and their chin.

Ask them to reach over their head with their left hand and pull their head forwards using their right fist as a pivot. Have them hold the fully stretched position for 2–5 seconds and then release.

## Variations

• Rather than holding the stretch, have your client use a gentle pulsing action, pulling and releasing rhythmically 10 times.

• Combine flexion with rotation by having them turn their head to look down to their right hip as they perform the traction. Reverse the action, looking down to the left.

## Points to note

By having your client use their fist as a pivot, the flexion force produced by their left hand (pulling down) opens the cervical spine, providing traction. The action of cervical flexion, keeping the chin tucked in towards the top of the sternum, encourages upper cervical motion. To increase the effectiveness of the action as your client pulls forwards with their left hand, ask them to also draw their hand upwards slightly, tending to slide (shear) the scalp tissues.

## Exercise 14.7 Neck bridge on block

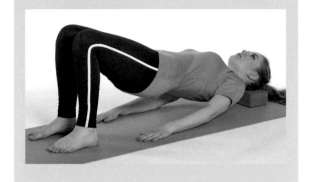

### Clinical scenario – stiff neck

Neck stiffness can occur through many causes and its treatment is by physiotherapy. As pain eases, however, exercise is useful both to remove stiffness and restore optimal head and neck alignment. Don't forget also that the neck has muscles and so just like any other body region it requires re-strengthening after injury.

When a client has neck pain it is common for them to develop a neck-forward posture. The chin tuck (Exercise 14.1) helps to correct this and often substantially relieves pain. It consists of a backward sliding action of the neck joints, and is progressed into skull rock standing back to wall (Exercise 14.2), which also involves flexing (opening) the upper cervical joints, which are often a main source of stiffness. Cervical rotation with overpressure (Exercise 14.5) eases stiffness to one side of the neck and also helps to restore symmetry to neck rotation. Begin building neck muscle strength using the isometric neck squeeze (Exercise 14.3) and when the muscles are stronger use neck bridge on block (Exercise 14.7) to develop greater strength relevant to contact sports especially.

### Aims and usage

To strengthen the cervical muscles prior to participation in contact sport

### Starting position and instructions

Begin with your client lying on the floor with their knees bent and feet hip-width apart. Place a firm foam pad (yoga block) or folded towel beneath their head, and have them keep their arms flat on the floor at an angle of 45 degrees to their body. They should tuck their chin in (head retraction) and press their head back into the block to lift their shoulders and upper back clear of the floor. Have them keep their hands and forearms on the floor for balance. They should aim to hold the upper position for 3–5 seconds and then release.

### Variations

• Once your client is in the lifted position, have them raise their arms from the floor to balance on their head and feet alone.
• Replace the yoga block with a rocker cushion (SITFIT®) or dome board (BOSU®) and perform the same action. As your client wobbles due to the unstable surface, ensure they keep their chest and shoulders parallel to the floor, avoiding any twisting action.

### Points to note

This action demands intense muscle work to the neck and shoulders to develop the high levels of strength and stability necessary for sports such as rugby, boxing and martial arts. It must only be practised when cervical alignment is optimal and when your client has mastered cervical stability exercise, such as the skull rock (Exercise 14.2) and isometric neck squeeze (Exercise 14.3).

# GLOSSARY

**Antagonist** The muscle that opposes the prime mover (*see* below) if it is contracted (e.g. the triceps, which relaxes if the biceps is contracted)

**Assistant movers (or secondary)** Muscles that may be able to help with the prime mover's action (*see* Prime mover) but are less effective than the prime mover.

**Basal metabolic rate (BMR)** The speed of chemical reactions when the body is at rest

**Biarticular** Muscle that crosses over two joints, e.g. the hamstrings, which attach from the seat bone (ischial tuberosity) to the top of the tibia. Since they cross both the hip and knee joints, they are capable of creating, or limiting, movement at both joints.

**Bursa** Fluid-filled fat pads and pouches around the joints that provide a cushion between bones and tendons and/or muscles around a joint, helping to reduce friction between the bones and allow free movement

**Closed skill** Occurs in a predictable (stable) environment, e.g. during a bench press when you are relatively isolated from changes in the environment as you are lying on a bench and only moving part of your body

**Consolidated oedema** Swelling that has become firm. When pressed, an impression of the finger tip is left behind (also called 'pitting oedema').

**Continuous skill** A skill that has no definite beginning or end but is repetitive in nature, e.g. walking or running

**Counterirritant** Relieving pain by introducing a second (intense) sensory stimulus

**Cytoskeleton** Connective tissue framework of the muscle

**Detraining** Failure to overload tissue sufficiently, resulting in loss of the benefits gained as part of the training adaptation

**Discrete skill** Skill that has a definite beginning and end, e.g. a sit-to-stand action. Once it is completed the skill has finished and you can go on to other things.

**Disuse atrophy** Muscle wasting due to lack of use

**Eburnation** Process during which the bone directly beneath fibrillation-damaged cartilage (*see* below) becomes smooth and shiny because the cartilage has begun to thin, reducing the distance between the bones

**Elasticity** The stretchiness of a material, or its ability to return to its original shape after a stress has deformed it

**Extensibility** The give in a material, or its ability to lengthen when subjected to stress

**Extracapsular** Ligament that is positioned outside the joint where it reinforces the joint capsule (e.g. the medial collateral ligament of the knee)

**Feedback** Process which tells a client how well a task was completed

**Feedforwards** Process which is predictive and provides information about what could happen in the future

**Fibrillation** Process during which the water content of cartilage increases due to chemical changes and the surface of the cartilage begins to fray. This is most noticeable in the areas at the side of the joint which are not weight-bearing. This can lead to osteoarthrosis (OA, *see* osteoarthrosis).

**Fibrin** Blood chemical involved in clotting

**Fibrous tissue** Non-contracting general soft tissue

**Graded exercise therapy (GET)** Physical activity that starts slowly and gradually increases throughout the treatment process

**Haemarthrosis** Bleeding into a joint. It can occur spontaneously or through injury.

**Haematoma** Blood clot

**Histamine** Chemical messenger involved in tissue healing which triggers the inflammatory response

**Hysteresis** Process by which ligament tissue weakens due to continued stretch over a prolonged period

**Inflammation** The first part of the tissue healing process. Inflammation is recognised by heat, redness, swelling and pain.

**Interneuron** Small connecting nerve lying between two longer nerves

**Intracapsular** Ligament that is positioned within the joint where it acts directly on the bone (e.g. the anterior cruciate ligament of the knee)

**Lag phase** Phase of injury rehabilitation during which the tissues begin to heal and a blood clot forms and shrinks, but it is still weak and easily disrupted by movement

**Length-tension relationship** The relationship between length of the muscle fibre and the force that the fibre produces at that length

**Leverage** Progresses an exercise by increasing the weight (load) of the object being lifted

**Lymph** Fluid found between body cells, also called interstitial fluid. Lymph flows within lymphatic vessels

**Metabolic rate** The speed of chemical reactions in the body

**Motor programme** Series of nerve (neural) commands which when initiated results in a single sequence of coordinated movements

**Movement dysfunction** Reduced quality of movement (e.g. limping)

**Multisensory** Process by which a number of types of cues are used (cues may be verbal, visual auditory or tactile in nature)

**Muscle inhibition** Wasting due to nerve impulses resulting from pain and swelling

**Myoglobin** An oxygen-binding protein

**Necrosis** The process during which injured tissue, starved of new blood which should bring with it oxygen and tissue nutrients, begins to die

**Non-steroidal anti-inflammatory drugs (NSAIDs)** Used to reduce pain and inflammation, especially in joint and muscle conditions, e.g. ibuprofen

**Oedema** The medical term for swelling, the accumulation of fluid beneath the skin (called 'edema' in the United States)

**Open skill** A skill performed within an unpredictable (unstable) environment, e.g. driving a car on the open road, which introduces distractions such as varying roads, other traffic and hazards

**Osteoblasts** Bone-forming cells

**Parallel processing** When you hear, see, feel, smell and taste several things at once

**Paratendonitis (or tenosynovitis)** Inflammation of the tendon sheath

**Part task training** Type of training that breaks down a complex movement or exercise into several component movements. Each individual movement can be practised and mastered and then the components put together.

**Phagocytosis** Process by which scavenging white blood cells (macrophages) remove dead cell material after injury

**Prime mover (or agonist)** Muscle which pulls to create a movement. Most muscles can take on this function, depending on the action required and the site of the muscle. If we take elbow flexion as an example, both biceps and brachialis can flex the elbow. In most circumstances the biceps is more effective and so acts as the prime mover, with the brachialis as the secondary mover.

**Progression** Process by which exercise must get harder to continue to sufficiently challenge the regenerating tissue

**Proprioception** Joint position sense

**Prostaglandin** Chemical messenger involved in tissue healing which causes vasodilation

**Regression** Process by which exercise is stopped and reintroduced at an easier level when your client reacts poorly, e.g. if they have a joint swelling or muscle ache

**Reversibility** Process by which athletes lose the effects of training when they stop working out ('use it or lose it')

**Sarcoplasm** Gel containing the fuel stores (glycogen) and enzymes important to muscle contraction

**Selective attention** A person's ability to pick out one stimulus (sound, vision, for example) within a field of numerous stimuli

**Serial skill** A number of individual discrete skills (*see above*) combined together as components of a larger skill

**Supercompensation** Process by which, when the body is overloaded, tissue breaks down at a microscopic level and rebuilds itself to become stronger

**Synapse** Junction between two nerves

**Tapering** Gradual reduction in training volume prior to a competition to give a physical and psychological break from the rigours of continuous training

**Tendonitis** Inflammation (swelling) of the tendon

**Tendinosis** Mild degeneration of the tendon substance

**Tenovaginitis** Roughening of the inner aspect of the sheath giving a grating (crepitus) sensation

**Trait** A persistent thought, emotion or behaviour pattern

**Vasodilation** Expansion or opening of blood vessels to increase blood flow in a tissue

**Whole task training** Method of training where you start with the whole complex action and accept that initially the performance of the action will be poor. Over time the action improves, as you remove those parts which are incorrect.

# REFERENCES

Borg, G. (1970) Perceived exertion as an indicator of somatic stress. *Scandinavian Journal of Rehabilitation Medicine* 2(2): 92–8

Bouchard, C., An, P., Rice, T., Skinner, J. S., Wilmore, J. H., Gagnon, J. (1999) Familial aggregation of VO2max response to exercise training: Results of the HERITAGE family study. *Journal of Applied Physiology* 87: 1003–8

Cochrane, D. J. (2011) Vibration exercise: The potential benefits. *International Journal of Sports Medicine* 32(2): 75–99

Cook, J. L., Khan, K. M. and Purdam, C. (2002) Achilles tendinopathy. *Manual Therapy* 7(3): 121–30

Costill, D. L., King, D. S., Thomas, R. and Hargreaves, M. (1985) Effects of reduced training on muscular power in swimmers. *Physician and Sports Medicine* 13(2): 94–101

Fiatrone, M. A. (1994) Exercise training and nutritional supplementation for physical frailty in very elderly people. *New England Journal of Medicine* 330: 1769

Houmard, J. A., Scott, B. K., Justice, C. L and Chenier, T. C. (1994) The effects of taper on performance in distance runners. *Medicine and Science in Sports and Exercise* 26: 624–31

Jarvinen, T. A. H., Jarvinen, T. L. N., Kaariainen, M., Aarimaa, V. et al (2007) Muscle injuries: Optimising recovery *Best Practice Research Clinical Rheumatology* 21(2): 317–31

Jarvinen, T. A. H., Jarvinen, T. L. N., Kaariainen, M., Kalimo, H. and Jarvinen, M. (2005) Muscle injuries: Biology and treatment. *American Journal of Sports Medicine* 33(5): 745–66

Lemmer, J. T., Hurlbut, D. E., Martel, G. F. and Tracy, B. L. (2000) Age and gender responses to strength training and detraining. *Medicine and Science in Sports and Exercise* 32: 1505–12

Norris, C. M. (2011) *Managing Sports Injuries* (Elsevier, Oxford)

Paterson, C. (1996) Measuring outcome in primary care: A patient-generated measure, MYMOP, compared to the SF-36 health survey. *British Medical Journal* 312: 1016–20

Persinger, R., Foster, C., Gibson, M. and Fater, D. (2004) Consistency of the talk test for exercise prescription. *Medicine and Science in Sports and Exercise* 36: 1632–6

Schmidt, R. A. and Lee, T. D. (2011) *Motor Control and Learning* (5th edition) (Human Kinetics, Champaign, Illinois)

Schmidt, R. A. and Wrisberg, C. A. (2008) *Motor Learning and Performance* (4th edition) (Human Kinetics, Champaign, Illinois)

Seidler, R. D., Noll, D. C. and Thiers, G. ( 2004) Feedforwards and feedback processes in motor control. *Neuroimage* 22(4): 1775–83

Sipala, S. and Suominen, H. (1995) Effects of strength and endurance training on thigh and leg muscle mass and composition in elderly women. *Journal of Applied Physiology* 78: 334

Weinberg, R. S. and Gould, D. (2007) *Foundations of Sport and Exercise Psychology* (4th edition) (Human Kinetics, Champaign, Illinois)

Williams, A. M., Davids, K. and Williams, J. G. (1999) *Visual Perception and Action in Sport* (Routledge, London)

Wilmore, J. H., Costill, D. L. and Kenney, W. L. (2008) *Physiology of Sport and Exercise* (4th edition) (Human Kinetics, Champaign, Illinois)

Zehr, E. P. and Sale, D. G. (1994) Ballistic movement: Muscle activation and neuromuscular adaptation. *Canadian Journal of Applied Physiology* 19(4): 363–78

# INDEX

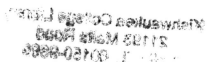